Fundamental Aspects of Caring for the Acutely Ill Adult

edited by
Pauleen Pratt

D0279871

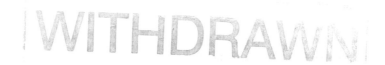

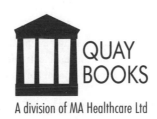

QUAY
BOOKS

A division of MA Healthcare Ltd

Quay Books Division, MA Healthcare Ltd, St Jude's Church, Dulwich Road, London
SE24 0PB

British Library Cataloguing-in-Publication Data
A catalogue record is available for this book

Printed in the UK by Cromwell Press Ltd, Aintree Avenue, Trowbridge, Wiltshire, BA14 0XB

Contents

Figures

Tables

To Dad and Bobby,
for their support, advice and love – always honest and
unconditional

Contributors

Pauleen Pratt, Consultant Nurse, Critical Care, University Hospitals Leicester NHS Trust

Susan Daykin, Specialist Nurse in Acute Pain, Leicester General Hospital, University Hospitals Leicester NHS Trust

John Kennedy, Specialist Nurse in Nutrition, Glenfield Hospital, University Hospitals Leicester NHS Trust

Caroline Barclay, Senior Nurse, Critical Care Outreach Service, University Hospitals Leicester NHS Trust

Alison Bricknell, Senior Staff Nurse, Critical Care Unit, Leicester Royal Infirmary, University Hospitals Leicester NHS Trust

Acknowledgements

I would like to thank Dr Neil Flint, whose advice and help in developing the format and detailing the contents, and suggestions for improvement, have been invaluable. His contributions have helped me to move forward and maintain a positive view when everything seemed impossible.

I would like to acknowledge the support and advice that Dr Apsara Leslie gave me in reading the final document; her friendship and professional support have been priceless.

Finally, I want to thank my colleagues for the support and advice they give me daily in my role as consultant nurse. They are honest, supportive and professional; I value and respect their advice. In particular, I would like to mention Caroline, Sarah, and Sanjay.

Preface

The hospital patient population is getting sicker and older. Increasingly, acutely ill patients, who were previously nursed in high-dependency areas, are now being cared for in general wards. Patients who are at risk of deterioration and are receiving advanced technical support, such as central venous line monitoring, high-flow oxygen, tracheostomy care and closer observations, are commonly being nursed within the busy ward setting. The ward nurse has to be aware of normal physiology and abnormal signs, in order to respond quickly, ensuring early detection of deterioration, systematic assessment and proactive management. This in turn will improve outcome by preventing further complications and, in some cases, death.

This book takes the nurse through the major systems of the body, relating physiology to practice. Each chapter follows a similar format, considering the observations that are recorded, the related anatomy and physiology, common diseases, treatments and interventions, and ending with a list of key learning points and revision questions. Additional learning points are highlighted within the text, and flow diagrams summarise other common areas, making the transfer to practice simple and concise. Aimed at the junior ward nurse, this book will help the nurse prioritise and identify key areas where deterioration is likely. It also highlights common problems that the general nurse is likely to encounter. The book is intended to be useful and user friendly across all specialties.

CHAPTER 1

Patient assessment

P Pratt

Nursing assessment of the acutely ill adult is of key importance to the ward nurse and needs to follow a systematic approach. It is important to consider all aspects of the patient's condition. You need to use all your senses as you approach and assess the patient. If you have not met the patient before, you will need to establish how he/she presents to you, and whether this is a stable state or whether there has been a change in the patient's condition.

Additional learning point
The 'End-of-the-bed test' is a key assessment of your patient. What do you see when you approach the patient; how does he/she look and respond?

At all times when assessing a patient's physiological state, it is important to maintain the patient's dignity by pulling the curtains around the bed or covering the patient with a sheet. The language you use to explain and reassure patients must be clear, so that they understand what they are being asked. Use open-ended questions and do not assume an answer. Regardless of any previous assessment, your assessment needs to include the following observations.

Consider the basics first

Is the patient maintaining his/her airway?

- Does the patient have a patent airway, or is he/she making sounds such as gurgling, snoring, or gasping, which may lead you to believe that he/she is unable to maintain an airway?

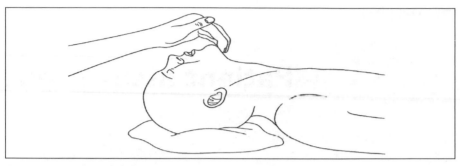

Figure 1.1: Head-tilt chin lift

If you feel that the patient is not maintaining an airway, you need to act immediately and ***call for help***. You then need to clear the airway using a head-tilt chin lift, as shown in *Figure 1.1*.

Is the patient breathing?

Factors to consider:

- Is the patient breathing?
- What is the respiratory rate?
- Is the breathing normal or abnormal, ie.are the accessory muscles being used?
- Does the patient have a wheeze?
- Is the patient able to talk in full sentences?
- What is the respiratory rate and what is the oxygen saturation?
- Is the patient on oxygen and, if so, what percentage (fractional concentration of oxygen in inspired air; FiO_2) is being delivered?

If the patient is finding it difficult to breathe, he/she will be very anxious and you need to have a calm manner while assessing and calling for help, so as to not distress the patient further.

Does the patient have a pulse and is the circulation adequate?

Factors to consider:

- Does the patient have a pulse?
- Is the pulse regular or irregular?

- Does it seem weak or thready?
- What is the blood pressure?
- Does the patient seem well perfused?
- Are the peripheries cold?
- Is the skin clammy or sweaty?
- Does the patient feel dizzy?

If any of these life-threatening abnormalities are found, actions to correct them must be undertaken as a matter of urgency. ***Call for senior help if in doubt.***

Once you have carried out a basic assessment of A (airway), B (breathing) and C (circulation) you can continue to further assess the patient's other systems. You need to work in a systematic way and recheck your findings if you are not sure of them. Sometimes you will be doing this assessment while completing other tasks around the patient. You need to use all your senses and ensure that you call for help if you suspect there are any abnormalities that you cannot manage.

Further assessment

Neurological function

As you approach the patient, consider the following:

- Does the patient look at you and respond?
- Does the patient talk to you when stimulated?
- Is the patient orientated in time and place?
- Does the patient respond only to pain?

A simple scale that can be used to assess conscious level is the AVPU (**A**lert, **V**oice, **P**ain, **U**nconscious) scale. The Glasgow coma scale (GCS) score is a well-recognised tool for assessing conscious level in more detail and is discussed further in *Chapter 4*.

If conscious level is altered, it is worth checking the blood glucose level, even if the patient is not known to have diabetes. Changes in conscious level, confusion and agitation are very important as they can be signs of more serious changes, and are often a reflection of developing sepsis or hypoxia. Initial assessment should include current neurological status, even if it is normal, and this should be documented so that trends can be monitored. Check the pupils. Are they equal and reacting? Are they small or large?

Another factor to be considered when assessing neurological function is the level of pain:

- Does the patient have pain?
- What kind of pain is it?
- Where is the pain?
- Has the patient received any analgesics recently?

Many pain-scoring tools are available and you need to be familiar with those in use locally. An example of a simple pain-scoring tool is shown in *Table 1.1*. Issues related to pain in the acutely ill patient are considered in more detail in *Chapter 8*.

Table 1.1: Pain-scoring tool

Score	0	1	2	3
	No pain at rest or on movement	No pain at rest; pain on movement	Pain at rest; worse on movement	Continuous pain at rest and on movement

> **Additional learning point**
> If concious level is significantly altered, the nurse should check a blood sugar even if the patient is not diabetic.

Gastrointestinal function

Factors to consider:

- Has the patient had surgery?
- Has the patient got a tender abdomen? Is it tense? Does it look red or mottled?
- Are there any wound or drain sites?
- How much drainage fluid is there? What does it look like?
- Does the patient feel nauseous?
- Is there a nasogastric tube in situ?
- Has the patient got a percutaneous endoscopic gastrostomy (PEG) or jejunostomy feeding tube in situ, and is the site clean or red?
- Is the patient eating and drinking or nil by mouth (NBM)?
- When did the patient last open his/her bowels? Was the stool normal or abnormal?

> **Additional learning points**
> Any abnormal findings need to be reassessed. Any actions/
> interventions must be followed by full reassessment to
> determine whether there has been an improvement
> or further deterioration.

Renal function

Factors to consider:

- Has the patient passed urine recently?
- What is the volume of urine passed?
- Is the urine concentrated? Does it smell?
- What does the urinalysis show?
- Does the patient have a urinary catheter in situ? Is it draining or could it be blocked?
- Have the urea and creatinine been checked recently? What are the results?
- Does the patient have a fluid balance chart? What is the overall balance? What has the balance been for the previous few days?

Fluid balance

The recording and interpretation of fluid balance in the acutely unwell adult is necessary to enable early detection of deterioration, which can then be acted upon. Fluid balance measurement is of key importance in the sick patient, and a fluid balance chart must be maintained and kept up to date. Measurement and documentation of input and output, as well as regular calculation of running totals and overall balance, are needed. The findings must be documented and accurate. Fluid charts vary, but they usually have an input side and an output side similar to that shown in the chart in *Figure 1.2*.

TIME	INPUT								OUTPUT						Balance
					Previous Input:								**Previous Output:**		**Balance:**
	Oral	Fluids IV Line	Drugs Infusion			PCA/ Epidural	NGT/ TPN	RT	Urine	Drains	Drains	Vomit/ NGT	Bowels	RT	
01															
02															
03															
04															
05															
06															
07															
08															
09															
10															
11															
12															
13															
14															
15															
16															
17															
18															
19															
20															
21															
22															
23															
24															
	Total Intake = _____ mls								Output (not including insensible loss) = _____ mls						

Figure 1.2: A typical fluid balance chart

Documentation

The initial assessment of the acutely ill adult is of key importance. It provides information that you need to consider in order to prioritise your actions and interventions. It allows you to give an informed summary of your concerns to the medical staff and ensures that timely and appropriate actions, which may prevent deterioration of your patient, are taken. Once you have assessed the patient, carried out any urgent interventions or called for senior help, you need to reassess the patient and decide whether the interventions you have carried out have improved the patient's condition. You must ensure that any assessment, findings and interventions are recorded, including the date, time and your name. The records you keep and the accuracy of the charts will make reassessment easier for you, and ensure that colleagues on other shifts have a full picture of the patient's general condition and are able to identify any trends in deterioration or improvement, and act on them.

Early warning systems

With the development of critical care outreach services following the publication of *Comprehensive Critical Care* (Department of Health, 2000) there has been much use of tools that use physiological parameters to generate scores that alert staff to a deterioration in the patient's condition. The recent National Confidential Enquiry into Patient Outcome and Death (NCEPOD) (2005) report highlights the need for such tools in facilitating early identification of patients at risk. The scores for individual physiological parameters are then added together to give an early warning score (EWS). If the EWS reaches a pre-agreed threshold value (trigger point), this will alert the practitioner completing the observations to inform a senior nurse or medical staff. This elevation in EWS score will also dictate an increase in the frequency of observations required by the patient. Appendix 1 shows an example of a trigger pathway.

It is important that nurses do not use the tool exclusively as it cannot do the job of experienced practitioners; the intuitive feeling that 'something is not right' should always be acted on, regardless of the EWS reaching a trigger point or not.

There are many different EWS systems in use and they all work on similar principles, namely the greater the deviation from 'normal', the greater the score generated. *Table 1.2* shows an example of an EWS tool. The first trigger point is a score of 4. Many early warning tools are incorporated into a basic chart that contains observations and fluid balance records. This tool uses normal blood pressure rather than current blood pressure, in order to take account of population variance. *Table 1.3* shows a grid that can be used to work out the EWS based on comparison of the patient's current and normal blood pressures.

Table 1.2: Modified early warning score (MEWS) tool

	Early warning score						
	3	2	1	0	1	2	3
HR(beats/min)		<40	40–50	51–100	101–110	111–129	≥130
RR (breaths/min)		≤8		9–14	15–20	21–29	≥30
Temperature (°C)		<35.0		35–38.4		≥38.5	
CNS				ALERT	VOICE	PAIN	UNCON
Urine total	NIL	<0.5ml/kg/h for 2 hours	<0.5ml/kg/h for 1 hour	<0.5ml/kg/h	>3ml/kg/h for 2 hours		
Blood pressure		See Table 1.3					

CNS = central nervous system; HR = heart rate, RR = respiratory rate

Table 1.3: Early warning scores generated from comparison of patient's normal and current systolic blood pressures

Patient's normal systolic blood pressure (mmHg)

CURRENT SYSTOLIC	200	190	180	170	160	150	140	130	120	110	100	90	80
200	0	0	0	1	1	2	2	2	3	3	4	5	5
190	0	0	0	1	1	1	1	2	2	3	3	4	5
180	0	0	0	0	0	0	1	1	2	2	3	3	4
170	1	1	0	0	0	0	1	1	2	2	3	3	4
160	1	1	1	0	0	0	0	1	2	2	2	2	3
150	1	1	1	1	0	0	0	0	1	1	1	2	2
140	2	2	1	1	1	0	0	0	0	0	1	1	2
130	2	2	2	1	1	1	0	0	0	1	1	1	1
120	2	2	2	2	2	1	0	0	0	0	2	2	2
110	3	3	2	2	1	1	1	0	0	0	0	0	0
100	3	3	3	3	2	2	2	1	1	0	0	0	0
90	4	4	4	3	3	3	2	2	2	2	1	0	0
80	4	4	4	4	3	3	3	2	2	2	2	1	0
70	4	4	4	4	4	3	3	3	2	2	2	2	1
60	5	5	5	5	4	4	3	3	3	3	3	2	1
50	5	5	5	5	5	5	5	5	4	4	4	3	2
40	6	6	6	6	6	6	6	6	5	5	5	4	3

Find patient's normal blood pressure across the top of the chart. Find current blood pressure down the left-hand side. The square where the two points meet shows the score generated. If scoring 4 on blood pressure, re-check measurement; if correct, summon assistance immediately.

Table 1.4 shows how to work out an EWS. Check which scoring system is in use in your local hospital.

Table 1.4: How to calculate an early warning score (EWS)

Patient observations in an 80kg man with normal blood pressure (BP) 140/70mmHg in clinic.

- Heart rate 105 beats/min
- Respiratory rate 17 breaths/min
- Temperature 36.8 °C
- Patient talking to you
- Urine passed in last hour 55ml
- Blood pressure 130/65mmHg

The scores run across the top of *Table 1.2* from zero to three.

Heart rate 105 falls in the 101–110 score box, so *scores 1 point.*

Respiratory rate 17 falls in the 15–20 score box, so *scores 1 point.*

Temperature 36.8 °C *scores 0.*

The patient is **alert** and **awake** and responds when you approach, so scores 0 for CNS.

In the past hour the patient has passed 55 ml of **urine**, so *scores 0* for urine output.

(The patient has passed >0.5ml/kg for that hour. Patients need to pass 50% of their body weight in urine, e.g. body weight 80kg = 40ml urine minimum per hour).

Blood pressure 130/65. Use *Table 1.3* to work out the score generated by this BP; the point where a score of 140 on the normal BP axis meets 130 on the current BP axis scores 0.

The total score for this set of observations is *2 points.*

After the total score has been calculated, there is a pathway to follow. Pathways tend to be agreed with individual wards, depending on case mix. An example of a modified EWS system flow pathway is shown in *Appendix 1.*

Summary

Your assessment of the patient will give you a baseline from which to work. The interventions you decide to implement and the actions you carry out can then be measured against any improvement or deterioration in your patient's condition.

If your patient is unwell, he/she will need close regular observation. All interventions, and the responses to these, need to be recorded. Early recognition and actions may prevent further deterioration. It will also ensure timely actions and may prevent serious organ dysfunction and possible death. As a nurse, your ability to monitor a patient, identify physiological abnormalities and respond in a timely way will save lives. Assessment of patients is a key skill when working in any acute ward area, and one that involves intuitive feelings as well as a good understanding of normal physiology. Communicating key concerns and documenting findings and actions will ensure safe and timely interventions for acutely ill adults in all ward areas.

Key learning points for *Chapter 1*

- Full assessment of the patient is the key to identifying acute problems and ensuring patient safety.
- Any assessment needs to be methodical and quick in the first instance.
- Remember the 'End-of-bed test'.
- Accurate recording of findings allows trends to be identified easily.
- Respiratory rate is a key observation and must be recorded as part of the general assessment.
- Early warning score (EWS) tools are useful, but a patient may still be unwell and not trigger a warning. Use your intuitive ability.
- If you report concerns to a senior member of staff and receive no support, go to the next most senior person.

Revision questions – patient assessment

I. Case study

Mr Peters is a 56-year old man who underwent a total hip replacement 2 days ago. He has no previous history of note and is normally fit and well. You have been allocated to care for him. When you approach him to prepare him for his morning care and complete his observations, you find him drowsy and responding to voice only. He feels warm to the touch and complains of wound pain.

What are your priorities as you assess him?

2. Work out early warning scores for the following patients

a. Jane Smith, 42 years old, weighed 65kg on admission. Her preoperative blood pressure was 130/80mmHg.

Heart rate	90 beats/min	Urine	70ml/h
Respiratory rate	16 breaths/min	Temperature	37.2 °C
Blood pressure	140/85mmHg	Neurological status	Alert

b. Bill Green, 52 years old, was admitted with pneumonia. He weighs 80kg and his blood pressure is not recorded in his notes.

Heart rate	110 beats/min	Urine	280ml in 9 hours
Respiratory rate	21 breaths/min	Temperature	38.2 °C
Blood pressure	130/60mmHg	Neurological status	Alert

c. Sally James, a 19-year-old student, is admitted with diabetic ketoacidosis. She weighs 90kg and her blood pressure was 160/70mmHg when she attended outpatients.

Respiratory rate	24 breaths/min	Urine	310ml in 12 hours
Temperature	37.5 °C	Neurological status	Responds to voice
Blood pressure	165/80mmHg	Heart rate	115 beats/min

You check Sally's observations one hour later. What is her score now?

Respiratory rate	20 breaths/min	Urine	40ml in last hour
Temperature	37.5 °C	Neurological status	Responds to voice
Blood pressure	165/80mmHg	Heart rate	98 beats/min

Answers on page 195

References

Department of Health (2000) *Comprehensive Critical Care: A review of adult critical care services.* DH, London

National Confidential Enquiry into Patient Outcome and Death (NCEPOD) (2005) *An Acute Problem?* NCEPOD, London

CHAPTER 2

Respiratory care

P Pratt and A Bricknell

Assessment and observations

History

A respiratory history needs to include the patient's normal respiratory state and how his/her current condition relates to that. You also need to consider the following:

- Does the patient smoke, how many and for how many years?
- Is the patient an ex-smoker?
- Does the patient have a cough normally and is it productive?
- What type of sputum is being expectorated?
- Is the patient on any relevant medication?
- Does the patient get breathless when exercising, dressing or at rest?
- How far can the patient walk before needing to rest due to shortness of breath?
- Does the patient sleep flat or with several pillows?
- Does the patient sleep in a chair?
- Does the patient have home oxygen or other respiratory support at home?
- Is there any relevant medical history of lung/breathing problems?

Assessment

Assessment of respiratory function is very important. You need to consider how well the patient is oxygenated and whether he/she has to work hard to maintain homeostasis. Remember also that respiratory rate is an indicator of more than just respiratory function. The need for oxygen must be assessed and a delivery method chosen to meet the patient's needs.

Early intervention must be ensured in a patient who is becoming hypoxic or responding to acid-base disturbances by an increase or decrease in respiratory rate. Tissue hypoxia will lead to irreversible damage and death if not treated quickly and effectively.

Assessment needs to include:

- Are the observations within normal ranges?
- Is the patient able to talk in full sentences?
- Is the patient positioning him/herself in such a way as to ease the shortness of breath?
- Is the patient using the accessory muscles to breathe?
- Does the patient look cyanosed?
- Is he/she breathing through pursed lips?
- Can he/she take a deep breath?
- Can the patient cough adequately?

Observations

Respiratory rate

This is a key observation that gives the nurse an indicator very early in a patient's deterioration that a problem is occurring. The respiratory rate should be recorded by holding the patient's wrist as if to take the pulse, and then observing chest movement for thirty seconds and doubling it to give the rate per minute. If the rate is very elevated or very slow, a full minute should be counted. The reason you need to appear to be recording the pulse is so that the patient does not become aware of you counting his/her breaths and does not voluntarily alter the rate. Remember to observe the pattern of breathing and the use of accessory muscles.

Oxygen saturation monitoring

Oxygen saturation (SpO_2) monitoring is carried out routinely in most clinical ward areas. It may even be seen as a replacement for respiratory rate, but it is not a replacement as it has several limitations and gives us different information from that obtained from respiratory rate.

A small probe is placed on the patient's ear or finger (*Figure 2.1*). It has two small light sources that pass through the tissue and are measured at the other side by a photocell. The system uses light absorbance measurements to determine concentrations of saturated haemoglobin.

Limits of oxygen saturation monitoring

Oxygen saturation measurements must be recorded and interpreted taking into account the amount of oxygen being received by the patient. A saturation measurement alone is of no use when assessing hypoxia.

Nail polish (particularly blue and black) and black henna may cause lower SpO_2 readings. It is always useful to remove any nail polish before using an oxygen saturation probe on the fingers.

Poor perfusion and vasoconstriction may make it difficult to obtain a reading and so restrict its use in very ill patients. It is important to check the site of the probe regularly as pressure sores can be caused in patients with poor circulation and those who are acutely unwell. Moving the sensor after each reading will help to prevent the development of pressure sores.

Carboxyhaemoglobin is picked up in the same way as oxyhaemoglobin, therefore oxygen saturation monitoring is of little use in patients with suspected carbon monoxide poisoning.

A patient who is anaemic may have normal oxygen saturations as all available haemoglobin is saturated; however, he/she may still be hypoxic.

Even though there are limits to the use of saturation monitoring, it is helpful in the ward setting and must be used in conjunction with full observation of a patient's other physiological parameters. The use of saturation monitoring may reduce the number of blood gas analyses that need to be performed. Oxygen saturation monitoring assists with early detection of hypoxia and is simple to use in a ward environment.

Additional learning point
Patients with normal oxygen saturations can still be acutely
unwell and hypoxic.

Blood gases

What do the results of arterial blood gas [ABG] analysis tell us? We have already considered oxygen saturations. As stated previously, SpO_2 tells us

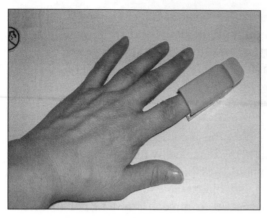

Figure 2.1: Oxygen saturation probe on finger

how much oxygen is attached to the available haemoglobin, but it does only tell us about oxygen levels, whereas ABG analysis tells us about acid-base balance. ABG results tell us the percentages of various gases present in the arterial circulation, including oxygen and carbon dioxide. ABG analysis also tells us about various other aspects of acid-base status of the blood, including the number of hydrogen ions, bicarbonate and lactate levels. Further information on this topic can be found in Woodrow (2003).

Basic interpretation of ABG results

Factors to consider:

- Was the patient receiving supplementary oxygen when the blood sample was taken, and what FiO_2 was being delivered?

- What is the PaO_2?
    - If PaO_2 is <10 kPa on air, the patient is hypoxic and requires supplementary oxygen to be delivered
    - If PaO_2 is >13 kPa on oxygen , it may be possible to decrease the supplementary oxygen being delivered

- What is the pH?
    - If pH is <7.35, this is an acidosis
    - If pH is >7.45, this is an alkalosis

- What is the serum bicarbonate and base excess (BE)? Is there a metabolic abnormality?
    - If the serum bicarbonate is <22 mmol/l and BE is >-2, there is a base deficit (metabolic acidosis)
    - If the serum bicarbonate is >26 mmol/l and BE >2, there is a positive BE (metabolic alkalosis)

■ What is the carbon dioxide partial pressure (PaCO$_2$)? Is there a respiratory abnormality?
   – If PaCO$_2$ is >6.1 kPa, the patient is retaining carbon dioxide (respiratory acidosis)
   – If PaCO$_2$ is <4.8 kPa, the patient is hyperventilating (respiratory alkalosis)

It is likely that the serum lactic acid level will also be recorded on the blood gas sample. A rise in lactic acid level above normal indicates tissue and cell hypoxia. Lactic acid is formed when there is not enough oxygen getting to the tissues.

> **Additional learning point**
> Lactic acid production is a sign of tissue and cell hypoxia.

Anatomy and physiology

An understanding of the respiratory system and how we breathe, in both mechanical and physiological terms, can help the nurse to recognise the signs shown by patients when they become unwell. This understanding will ensure that the nurse prioritises the interventions and actions to improve oxygenation and respiratory function while relieving patient distress and anxiety. *Figure 2.2* shows the basic structure of the respiratory system.

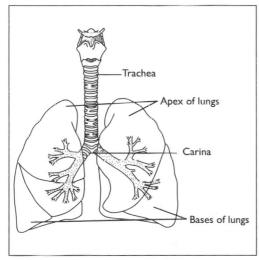

Figure 2.2: Basic structure of the respiratory system

Anatomy

The trachea

The trachea is a pipe-like structure that passes from the pharynx down into the lobes of the right and left lung. It divides into the right and left primary bronchi, where there is an internal ridge called the carina. The mucous membrane of the carina is one of the most sensitive areas of the airway for triggering a cough reflex.

The inner surface of the trachea (epithelium) consists of ciliated columnar cells and goblet cells. The epithelium provides the same protection against dust as does the membrane lining the nasal cavity and larynx.

Additional learning point
Suction down a tracheostomy tube or airway can cause trauma to the tracheal membrane, so caution is required.

The lungs

Human beings have two lungs. The right lung has three lobes (upper, middle and lower) and the left lung has two lobes (upper and lower). The heart and other structures in the mediastinum separate the lobes from each other. The mediastinum separates the thoracic cavity into two anatomically distinct chambers. Because of these two separate chambers, if trauma causes one lung to collapse the other may remain expanded. Two layers of serous membrane, collectively called the pleural membrane, enclose and protect the lung.

Each segment of the lung has many small compartments called lobules. Each lobule is wrapped in elastic connective tissue and contains a lymphatic vessel, an arteriole, a venule and a branch from a terminal bronchiole. Terminal bronchioles subdivide into microscopic branches called respiratory bronchioles. As the respiratory bronchioles penetrate more deeply into the lungs, they in turn subdivide into alveolar ducts.

The alveoli

Around the circumference of the alveolar ducts are numerous alveoli and alveolar sacs. An alveolus is a cup-shaped bulb lined with simple epithelium and supported by a thin elastic membrane. Alveolar sacs comprise two or more alveoli that share a common opening. The alveolar walls consist of two types of alveolar epithelial cells: type 1 and type 2. The thin type 1 cells form the area where gas exchange takes place. Type 2 cells secrete surfactant, which keeps the alveolar cells moist. Around the alveoli is a discrete capillary network, with the walls of each capillary consisting of a single layer of cells.

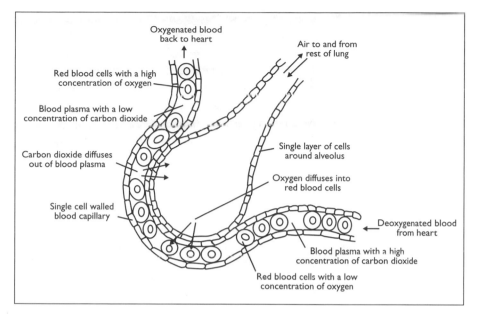

Figure 2.3: Gaseous exchange in the alveoli of the lungs

Exchange of the two main respiratory gases, oxygen and carbon dioxide, between the lungs and blood takes place by diffusion across the alveolar and capillary walls *(Figure 2.3)*. The layer through which the respiratory gases diffuse is known as the alveolar–capillary membrane. This membrane is very thin and allows for rapid diffusion of respiratory gases. It has been estimated that the lungs contain 300 million alveoli, providing a surface area of around 70m² for the exchange of gases.

Lung volumes and capacities

In clinical practice, the word ventilation means one inspiration and one expiration. The healthy adult averages twelve ventilations in a minute and moves about six litres of air per minute into and out of the lungs while at rest. A lower than normal volume of air exchange is usually a sign of pulmonary malfunction. The equipment commonly used to measure the volume of air exchanged during breathing, and the rate of ventilation, is termed a spirometer.

Additional learning point
Peak flow is measured in the ward area to obtain a baseline value for the patient's maximum expired forced volume. This enables the effect of treatment to be monitored, and improvements or deteriorations in the underlying condition of patients with obstructive airways diseases to be identified.

Various lung volumes can be measured. For each volume, we will consider the normal volume and what specifically it is measuring. During quiet breathing in the average adult, 500ml of air moves in and then out of the airways with each inspiration and expiration. This is the volume of one breath and is called the tidal volume (V_T). V_T varies considerably from person to person, and in the same person at different times. In an average adult, about 70% (350ml) of V_T reaches the respiratory bronchioles, alveolar ducts, alveolar sacs and alveoli, and hence participates in gas exchange. The other 30% (150ml) remains in the air spaces of the nose, pharynx, larynx, trachea, bronchi, bronchioles and terminal bronchioles; these areas are known collectively as the anatomical dead space.

Additional learning point
In a patient with a tracheostomy, part of the anatomical dead space is bypassed and hence each breath tidal volume can be smaller but still ventilate the alveoli adequately.

The total volume of air taken in during one minute is called the minute volume (MV) or minute ventilation. It is calculated by multiplying V_T by the normal breathing rate per minute.

$$
\begin{aligned}
\text{Average MV} \quad &= \quad \text{500ml x 12 respirations per minute} \\
&= \quad \text{6000ml/min} \\
&= \quad \text{6 litres/min}
\end{aligned}
$$

Not all of the MV can be used in gas exchange, however, because some of it remains in the anatomical dead space. The alveolar ventilation rate (AVR) is the volume of air per minute that reaches the alveoli.

In the above example:

$$AVR = 350\text{ml} \times 12 \text{ respirations per minute}$$
$$= 4200 \text{ ml/min}$$
$$= 4.2 \text{ litres/min}$$

During strenuous breathing, other lung volumes come into play. In general these volumes are larger in males, taller persons and younger adults, and smaller in females, shorter persons and elderly people. Various disorders may also be diagnosed by comparison of actual and predicted normal values for gender, height and age.

A person can inspire a great deal more than 500ml air by taking a very deep breath. This additional inhaled air is called the inspiratory reserve volume. It is about 2500ml above the 500ml V_T – a total of 3000ml. Even more air can be inhaled if inspiration follows forced expiration. If a person inhales normally and then exhales as forcibly as possible, he/she should be able to push out 1500ml of air in addition to the 500ml V_T. If a person inhales as much air as possible and then blows out until he/she can blow no more, this volume is called the forced vital capacity (FVC). The extra 1500ml that is exhaled is called the expiratory reserve volume (ERV). Inspiration is recorded as an upward deflection and expiration as a downward deflection.

Even after the ERV is expelled, a considerable volume of air remains in the lungs because the alveoli remain lightly inflated, and some air remains in the non-collapsible airways. This volume, which cannot be measured by spirometry, is called the functional residual capacity (FRC) and amounts to about 1200ml.

Additional learning point

When positive end-expiratory pressure (PEEP) is applied to a patient's breathing system during continuous positive airways pressure (CPAP) or mechanical ventilation, the functional residual capacity (FRC) is increased. A greater volume of air can therefore be utilised for gas exchange.

Lung capacities are combinations of specific lung volumes. Inspiratory capacity (the total inspiratory ability of the lungs) is the sum of V_T plus inspiratory reserve volume (3000ml). FRC is the sum of residual volume plus ERV (3000ml). Vital capacity (VC) is the sum of inspiratory reserve volume, V_T and ERV (4500ml). Finally, total lung capacity is the sum of all volumes (6000ml). *Table 2.1* summarises these volumes.

Nervous control of breathing

Muscles in the thoracic cavity relax and contract under the control of nerve impulses from the medulla and the pons in the brain.

Additional learning point

In a patient with a head injury or stroke, respiration may be affected through involvement of the respiratory centre. Respiratory rate and pattern may be altered, but the patient does not have any lung problems.

The respiratory centre comprises:

* The inspiratory centre (medulla)
* The expiratory centre (medulla)
* The pneumotactic centre (pons)
* The apnoeic centre (medulla).

Impulses from the respiratory centre are tonic and hence do not require a stimulus for generation. Impulses from the inspiratory centre of the medulla pass along the phrenic nerve to the diaphragm, and from the intercostal nerve to the external intercostal muscles. The pneumotactic centre in the pons also receives impulses from the inspiratory centre and passes impulses to the expiratory centre, thereby allowing expiration.

A person can consciously control breathing as the cerebral cortex can override the inspiratory centre.

Chemical control of breathing

Peripheral and central sensory nerve receptors, called chemoreceptors, detect and respond to changes in the level of carbon dioxide in the blood. They then send impulses to the inspiratory centre to increase or decrease respiratory rate to maintain homeostasis. The respiratory system maintains a balance of carbon dioxide and oxygen levels within the normal range.

Carbon dioxide is the main influencing chemical that controls respiratory rate. Carbon dioxide affects the level of hydrogen ions (H^+), which are formed by the breakdown of carbonic acid from carbon dioxide and water in the lungs. An increase in the level of carbon dioxide in the blood is reflected by an increase in H^+. The chemoreceptors in the walls of the main blood vessels monitor carbon dioxide levels. If they detect an increase in carbon monoxide levels (hypercapnia), the medulla is stimulated to increase respiratory rate so that more carbon dioxide is exhaled and the elevated level is corrected. An increased respiratory rate without hypoxia should be further examined as it may indicate more complex acid-base disorders.

If the chemoreceptors detect a fall in carbon dioxide level below a baseline, the inspiratory centre is stimulated, causing a fall in respiration rate. However, if the carbon dioxide falls too low, stimulation can cease and apnoea may occur.

Gas exchange

Respiration is the exchange of oxygen and carbon dioxide between air in the alveoli of the lungs and blood in the pulmonary capillaries. It results in the conversion of deoxygenated blood coming from the heart to oxygenated blood returning to the heart. During inspiration, atmospheric air containing 21% oxygen enters the alveoli, and during expiration carbon dioxide is exhaled into the atmosphere. Deoxygenated blood is pumped from the right ventricle through the pulmonary arteries into the pulmonary capillaries that surround the alveoli. The surface area of capillaries around the alveoli in the lungs is very large.

Additional learning point

An increased respiratory rate without hypoxia should be further examined as it may indicate more complex acid base disorders.

The PO_2 of alveolar gas is 14kPa. In a person at rest, the PO_2 of deoxygenated blood entering the pulmonary capillaries is about 5.3kPa. If the person has been exercising, it will be even lower. Because of the difference in PO_2 there is a net diffusion of oxygen from the alveoli into the deoxygenated blood until equilibrium is reached. The PO_2 of the now oxygenated blood increases to 14kPa. Because blood leaving the capillaries near the alveoli mixes with a small volume of blood that has not flowed close to the alveoli, the PO_2 of blood in the pulmonary veins is about 13.3kPa.

While oxygen diffuses from the alveoli into deoxygenated blood, there is a net diffusion of carbon dioxide in the opposite direction. The PCO_2 of deoxygenated blood is 6.1kPa in a resting person, whereas the PCO_2 of alveolar gas is 0.04kPa. Because of this difference, carbon dioxide diffuses from deoxygenated blood into the alveoli until the PCO_2 of the blood decreases to 5.3kPa, ie. the PCO_2 of fully oxygenated blood. *Figure 2.6* summarises the change in partial pressure during inspiration and expiration.

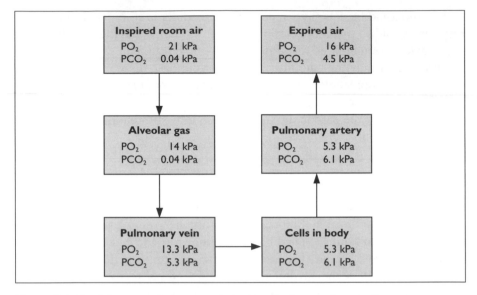

Figure 2.6: Partial pressure changes during inspiration and expiration

Elevation of the carbon dioxide level in the blood causes the stimulation of chemoreceptors in the aorta and the carotid bodies, which leads to changes in respiratory rate; these chemoreceptors are sensitive to PCO_2 and PO_2 and are called the peripheral chemoreceptors. There are also central chemoreceptors in the medulla that respond to changes in PCO_2. Peripheral chemoreceptors are not particularly sensitive and a large rise in PCO_2 is needed to stimulate them.

Central chemoreceptors are located on the ventral surface of the medulla and are exposed to cerebrospinal fluid (CSF); they respond to changes in the pH of the CSF. A rise in carbon dioxide level, and hence $PaCO_2$, will lead to a fall in pH, which in turn causes the respiratory rate to rise. If $PaCO_2$ falls and pH rises, then respiratory rate will fall. This effect forms part of the negative feedback loop that maintains homeostasis.

Hypoxic respiratory drive

In a very small group of patients who have a stable but elevated PCO_2 due to chronic respiratory disease, the respiratory centres in the brain reset themselves. In the normal adult without chronic respiratory disease small changes in arterial PCO_2 will produce rapid changes in respiratory rate, in an attempt to stabilise PCO_2. However, in the patient with chronic respiratory disease, if PCO_2 remains high for a period of time the activity of the choroid plexus will reset the system to accept a higher PCO_2 as its norm, but the hypoxic drive in the peripheral chemoreceptors will be maintained.

> **Additional learning points**
> If a patient has a history of COPD, oxygen should be given but with
> caution, and regular observations of respiratory rate and conscious level
> should be carried out after each increase in FiO_2.
> It is important to remember that there is a greater chance of hypoxia
> resulting in death than a patient becoming apnoeic due to the delivery of
> too much oxygen. Close observation, however, is essential and there is no
> room for complacency in this group of patients.

Oxygen carriage and delivery

Oxygen is mostly carried in the blood bound to haemoglobin in red blood
cells; the saturation of the haemoglobin is measured by pulse oximetry.
Each haemoglobin molecule can carry up to four oxygen molecules. A small
amount of oxygen is also carried dissolved in the plasma. This small fraction
is measured by blood gas analysis. These two portions added together equal
the oxygen content of the blood.

Oxygen delivery is the product of the oxygen content of the blood and
cardiac output. Cardiac output is discussed further in *Chapter 3*.

The ability of the body to:

* Maintain respiratory function
* Carry oxygen in the blood
* Maintain an adequate cardiac output.

are vital components for life. Many treatments discussed in this book are
related to optimising these important functions.

Respiratory diseases

Respiratory failure

Respiratory failure is defined as an inability of the pulmonary system
to maintain adequate gas exchange in the alveoli. This may be caused

Key problems

Physiotherapy and simple measures, such as good positioning and adequate hydration, will aid expectoration. Supporting abdominal wounds and adequate and effective pain relief will also help to optimise the patient's potential for clearing secretions. The removal of secretions by an effective cough can be difficult to maintain if the patient is becoming tired. Often, the reason that patients are intubated and ventilated is that they are not able to clear their secretions and therefore hypoxia worsens.

Chronic obstructive pulmonary disease (COPD)

COPD is a collective name for three disorders: emphysema, chronic bronchitis and chronic asthma. These are obstructive lung diseases which develop as chronic, slowly progressive disorders characterised by a gradual increase in airflow obstruction.

Risk factors

- Smoking
- Infection
- Increasing age
- Allergy
- Air pollution
- Genetic risk
- Coal mining.

Signs and symptoms

- Shortness of breath on exertion
- Chronic cough
- Wheeze
- Chronic excessive secretions.

Key problems

Patients with COPD are prone to infections and acute exacerbation of these chronic disorders, with worsening symptoms and decreasing functional ability, for which they will often require multiple hospital admissions. This group of patients requires close observation, and treatment aims include early detection of new infections or worsening oxygenation. If these patients are intubated and ventilated, their prognosis can be very poor and they are often on the critical care unit for extended periods of time. It is important to prevent deterioration, although often this may not be possible in the end stages of the disease.

Acute asthma

Acute asthma is defined as a reversible inflammatory airway disease that results in bronchoconstriction and airway obstruction.

Risk factors

- Allergy
- Infection
- Smoking
- Stress.

Signs and symptoms

- Wheeze
- Cough
- Shortness of breath
- Tightness in chest
- Tachycardia
- Anxiety
- Hyperinflation of the chest
- Use of accessory muscles in breathing
- Elevated carbon dioxide in the later stages
- Hypoxia
- Unable to talk in full sentences.

Key problems

The patient with acute asthma who is not treated will be at high risk of respiratory collapse due to an inability to exhale and over-inflation of the chest. Spontaneous pneumothorax and increased respiratory dysfunction are common. The patient will often be very scared, restless and agitated, and will need close observation and reassurance.

Pulmonary embolism

Pulmonary embolism is defined as the obstruction of one of the pulmonary arteries by an embolism.

Risk factors

- Deep vein thrombosis
- Postoperative status
- Immobility
- Coagulation disorders
- Trauma
- Atrial fibrillation.

Signs and symptoms

- Fall in oxygen and carbon dioxide levels on blood gas analysis
- Chest pain
- Shortness of breath
- General deterioration in condition without obvious cause
- Cough
- Risk of cardiac arrest.

Key problems

The patient will often feel very anxious, and be short of breath and in pain. Treatments may be ineffective and slow to work. Diagnosis is often difficult and false positives and negatives can be obtained from some investigations.

Pneumothorax

Pneumothorax is defined as the spontaneous occurrence of air in the pleural space due to disease or trauma. It is important to determine the cause of the pneumothorax so that it can be treated after initial management of the pneumothorax. A simple pneumothorax will leak air into the pleural space and decompress the lung, leading to hypoxia, and can be treated after the cause has been confirmed by X-ray. A tension pneumothorax, however, must be treated as an emergency as air cannot leave the pleural space and the lung and right ventricle become compressed, leading to a reduction in cardiac output and possible cardiac arrest.

Risk factors

- Trauma
- Over-dilated alveoli
- Lung disease.

Signs and symptoms

- Hypoxia
- Shortness of breath
- Chest pain
- Decreased chest movement.

Key problems

The patient with a pneumothorax is at risk of developing a tension pneumothorax. This occurs when the air in the pleural space is under pressure, and can lead to lung collapse and cardiac shift. This causes a reduction in cardiac output and may lead to cardiac arrest. The patient will usually require an underwater seal drain to remove the air and allow the chest to re-inflate.

Treatments and interventions

Basics

- Positioning: Correct positioning of the patient will ensure maximum lung expansion with minimum effort. Sitting up in a chair is best mechanically for chest movement; also, the movement to the chair will act as physiotherapy. When in a chair the patient should be well supported; a table positioned in front of the patient for him/her to rest on may also help. If patients are not well enough to sit out of bed, they should be sat well up in bed supported by pillows – not slumped down.

- Cough: Encouraging coughing will assist in clearing secretions and help to reduce the risk of respiratory failure. Reminding the patient to cough and expectorate whenever you are passing will help to maximise sputum clearance. If a patient is unable to cough, then nasopharyngeal suctioning may be required to stimulate a cough and clear secretions.

- Deep breathing: Getting the patient to breathe deeply will ensure expansion of the lung bases. This will not only help to prevent and treat alveolar collapse, but will also assist in producing a good cough.

- Physiotherapy: Asking the physiotherapist to assess a patient will ensure optimisation of respiratory function, as these health professionals are highly skilled in breathing exercises and optimising secretion clearance. They are also skilled in the use of various devices to ensure lung expansion and maintenance of secretion clearance.

- Pain relief: Patients who have had surgery may not be able to breathe deeply or cough because of pain; managing their pain is therefore important in preventing respiratory failure and maximising their ability to adequately ventilate the lungs. Patients should be asked to breathe deeply and cough and give an assessment of the pain they experience while doing these exercises. Any pain should be treated by the administration of an appropriate prescribed analgesic, and the nurse should ensure that this is administered as prescribed.

- Reassurance: A patient who is short of breath will be very anxious and may, in extreme cases, express a fear of dying because of this. The nurse needs to reassure the patient and explain the benefits of the treatment being given in order to alleviate the patient's distress. Some patients may benefit from relaxation techniques; although sedation should ideally be avoided, in some cases mild drug therapy may be indicated, provided that it does not compromise respiratory drive.

Oxygen therapy

Oxygen is a drug and should be prescribed for individual patients as required. It is also a gas that supports combustion and is therefore a fire hazard. It is very dry when delivered from a source in a ward and can lead to drying of the mucus in the airways; patients receiving high flow rates and high percentages of oxygen therefore require extra humidification.

Caution is often advised if a patient is thought to rely on a hypoxic drive and has a raised but stable carbon dioxide level. A patient with a hypoxic drive is stimulated to breathe by low oxygen levels in the blood, as the chemoreceptors have become adjusted to elevated carbon dioxide levels and do not respond in the normal way. Hence a patient receiving supplementary oxygen will detect a rise in PO_2 and thus stop breathing. A patient with a history of COPD should be observed for signs of drowsiness and fall in respiratory rate when commencing oxygen therapy and after any increase in FiO_2.

It is also important to note that although hypoxia must be treated, high concentrations of oxygen over long periods of time can be toxic to

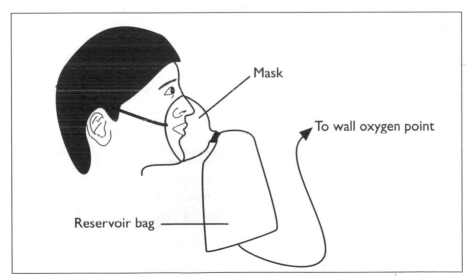

Figure 2.7: Non-rebreathe oxygen mask reservoir

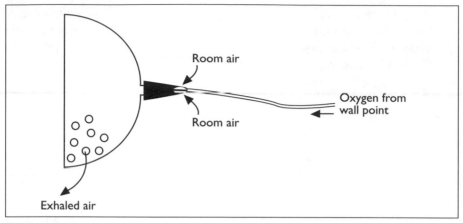

Room air

Oxygen from wall point

Room air

Exhaled air

Figure 2.8: Example of a Venturi oxygen mask

lung tissue; patients on high oxygen concentrations should therefore be weaned onto lower concentrations whenever possible, while maintaining adequate oxygenation.

Methods of oxygen administration

There is a variety of systems for delivering oxygen within the ward area. Some of these are discussed below.

- Nasal cannulae: These are simple and fit around the patient's head; they have two small prongs which fit into the nose, through which oxygen is delivered. They connect to a wall oxygen point flow meter and can deliver a maximum of 35% FiO_2. Oxygen flow should not be greater than 4 litres/min, otherwise the patient may develop mucosal burning. Nasal cannulae are useful in patients who cannot tolerate a face mask and who need a small amount of oxygen to maintain adequate oxygenation.

- Face mask (Hudson) with or without a reservoir: This mask covers the mouth and nose, and FiO_2 can be increased to around 90% if a non-rebreathe reservoir is attached *(Figure 2.7)*. The limiting factor will be the patient's peak inspiratory flow, which increases when respiratory rate and respiratory effort increase. In this case the patient needs to be given high-flow oxygen (see later).

- Venturi mask: This mask delivers a set FiO_2 and is used in patients where tight control of the oxygen delivered must be assured. It will indicate the flow rate that needs to be set off the wall flow meter in order to deliver the set FiO₂ *(Figure 2.8)*.

Humidification

In the well adult, air passes over the cilia and mucous membranes of the upper airways via the nose during inspiration. In the acutely unwell adult, mouth breathing is common and the mucous membranes are bypassed, leading to drying of the airways. During expiration, approximately 200ml of water is lost in the expired air over a 24-hour period. The volume of water lost in this way increases in the patient with an elevated respiratory rate, hence supplementary humidification is needed in addition to adequate oral hydration.

Humidification can be achieved by means of cold or warm water systems. The warm water system includes a heating device *(Figure 2.9)*, which warms the inspired air that passes to the patient, and the increase in temperature of the gas increases its ability to carry water molecules. The water molecules carried in heated systems are smaller than those carried in cold water systems, hence heated systems deliver humidification further into the respiratory tract.

When a patient is receiving supplementary oxygen and humidification, the nurse should check the oxygen flow rate and humidifier settings when completing patient observations. This will ensure that the humidified air is the correct temperature and the reservoir is filled with water.

As the air cools, some of the water vapour will condense and may sit in the tubing; this should be emptied at regular intervals as it will prevent the flow of gas and is a potential source of infection. Breathing cold, dry air directly into the trachea can cause paralysis of the cilia and crusting of secretions, which may lead to infection, obstruction and other complications (Casey, 1989). Viscous mucus increases:

* Risk of infection
* Risk of airway encrustation/obstruction

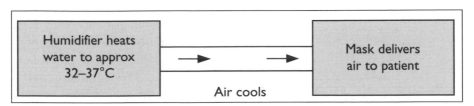

Figure 2.9: Principle of a heated humidification system

- Airway resistance and work of breathing
- Surfactant dysfunction
- Risk of infection.

Methods of humidification

■ Warm water humidification: In this method, gas is driven over or through a heated water reservoir. This airflow absorbs water, which is carried as vapour and is then inspired by the patient. The thermostat is set at a temperature of 32–37°C. The air cools as it passes along the tubing, reaching the patient at approximately 35°C. Because of the differing equipment available, the nurse should check details regarding the set temperature with the manufacturer. This type of humidification is ideal for patients with thick, sticky secretions.

■ Cold water humidification: This method delivers partially humidified gas, and is commonly available within the ward setting. This is ideal for patients who are expectorating secretions well, and require only slight humidity. Because the air is cold, its ability to carry water molecules is reduced.

■ Aerosol generator (nebuliser): In this method, a jet of gas at high pressure passes near a water reservoir and draws water up a tube by a suction effect (the Venturi effect). It then hits a baffle and is broken into micro-droplets. Saline nebulisers are recommended 2–4 hourly for patients with excessive thick, crusting secretions.

High-flow oxygen therapy

This system can deliver between 30% and 100% FiO$_2$, and does this at a 'high flow' in order to meet the peak inspiratory demand of the patient. In patients with high respiratory rates and poor SpO$_2$, this is the system of choice. *Figure 2.10* summarises the set-up of a high-flow oxygen delivery system.

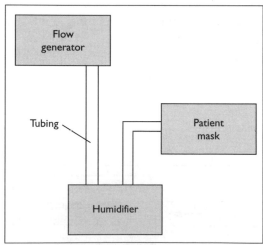

Figure 2.10: Set-up of a high-flow oxygen delivery system

Chest tubes and drainage systems

A chest tube is inserted to remove air or fluid from the pleural cavity. Insertion of a chest tube may be required following surgery, disease or injury. The position of the drainage tube will depend on the substance that is to be drained. If an effusion is to be drained the tube is likely to be more basally placed, and if air is to be drained the tube is likely to be placed nearer the apex. The tube is then attached to an underwater drainage system.

Tube insertion

The drain may be inserted intraoperatively if it is required following a surgical procedure, or on a ward for drainage of a pneumothorax (air in the pleural cavity) or pleural effusion. Blood (haemothorax) and pus (empyema) can also be drained using a chest tube.

If the drain is inserted on the ward, the nurse needs to be aware of local policy. The following list highlights important aspects of care:

* Reassurance for the patient
* Comfortable positioning of the patient for drainage tube insertion and expansion of the rib cage
* Adequate analgesia for the procedure and afterwards
* Preparation of the drainage system
* Ongoing monitoring of drainage
* Monitoring of patient's vital signs
* Care of the chest tube site
* Availability of drain clamps in case of emergency.

Underwater seal drainage system

The drainage tube is attached to an underwater seal drain *(Figure 2.11)*. A Heimlich valve can also be used and is commonly employed in patients who are more mobile but still need a drainage system. The valve works by allowing fluid and air to pass in one direction only.

The system works by gravity; positive pressure and suction can also be added. Because it works by gravity, the drainage system must always be positioned below the level of the patient. Air passes from a higher level to a lower level; if the system is raised higher than the patient, fluid and air can pass back into the pleural cavity, compromising the patient and increasing the risk of infection.

Nursing care of the patient with a chest drain in situ

Observe the system to ensure that it is patent and working by looking for:

- Air bubbling into the drain (this should reduce and stop when the lung is fully inflated)
- Fluid in the drainage tube moving up and down with respiration
- Increasing volume of fluid collecting in the drainage bottle (this should be checked and recorded at least once every shift).

Ensure that clamps are available for clamping the chest drainage tube. It is important to avoid clamping the drainage tube unless an emergency has occurred, eg. the bottle has come disconnected or a large volume has drained and you are instructed to clamp the tube. The only reason to clamp a tube electively is to change the bottle or to check that lung expansion is maintained before removal of the tube.

The drain site and dressing should be checked at least daily. If the site looks red or dirty, or pus is visible, a swab should be sent for culture. The nurse should also observe the position of the tube and confirm that it is still the correct length, ie. the same length as when first inserted, and that there are no holes on the part of the tube external to the skin. If holes are seen in the tube external to the skin, or the tube is not inserted as far as it was initially, the medical staff should be informed to review the position.

Adequate pain relief must be administered. Some patients will feel better knowing that the drain has improved their breathing, but others may still feel very uncomfortable and the drain may be causing them pain. Each patient's needs regarding analgesia are different.

Details of the drainage fluid should be recorded at regular intervals, including the type of drainage in the bottle. Any change in colour or fresh blood in the fluid should be reported to a senior member of staff.

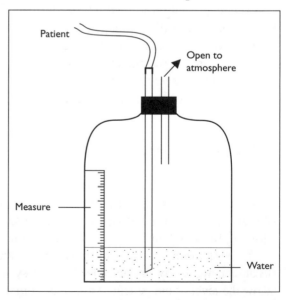

Figure 2.11: Set-up of an underwater seal drainage system

The drainage bottle must be changed when it becomes full. The bottle should be kept upright at all times, ensuring that the drainage tube is under water.

Removal of the tube is generally done by an experienced nurse and includes reassuring the patient, removal of the drain after removing the suture, and closing the wound by pulling the purse suture tight. Check with your local guideline as to who should carry out drain removal on your ward.

Drugs

Nebulised drugs

These are drugs given as a mist of tiny droplets, which are inhaled and delivered deep into the airways. Nebulised drugs are given in the acute phase of an illness, as drugs administered in this way have a greater effect than those given by inhaler.

Drugs commonly given by nebulisation include:

- Bronchodilators, such as salbutamol, which work on the beta-2 receptors causing smooth muscle in the bronchi to relax and so open the airways, easing respiratory effort.
- Anticholinergics, such as ipratropium, which promote relaxation of smooth muscle and reduce secretions.

Nebulised salbutamol and ipratropium can have side-effects, including tachycardia and tremor.

Intravenous drugs

Aminophylline may be given as an intravenous infusion in acutely unwell patients with respiratory failure. It is a phosphodiesterase inhibitor and relaxes smooth muscle. This drug has many adverse effects and the nurse needs to be familiar with these when caring for a patient receiving an aminophylline infusion. The side-effects include:

- Tachycardia
- Arrhythmias

- Nausea
- Abdominal pain
- Convulsions.

Antibiotics will be given to patients with a suspected bacterial infection. It is usual for such patients to be prescribed a broad-spectrum antibiotic that will be effective against a variety of bacterial infections. A different antibiotic is given for a community-acquired infection compared with a hospital-acquired infection, and the nurse should be aware of local prescribing policy. As soon as possible, the nurse should send a sputum sample for microbiology, culture and sensitivity to ensure that the patient is on the correct treatment. Ideally, this sample should be sent before antibiotic treatment commences.

Advanced respiratory support

Continuous positive airways pressure (CPAP)

CPAP is a system in which a set FiO_2 is delivered with a positive end-expiratory pressure (PEEP) in the system. PEEP increases the functional residual capacity and improves oxygenation while reducing the work of breathing. *Appendix 2* shows a pathway that can be used to help the practitioner determine whether CPAP is indicated.

Patients need close observation when undergoing CPAP as they have a tight-fitting mask on and may become distressed. Other potential complications are shown in *Table 2.2*.

Contraindications to non-invasive CPAP

- Hypoventilation (respiratory rate <8 breaths/min)
- Reduction in conscious state/risk of aspiration
- Acute myocardial infarction
- Hypotension (systolic blood pressure <80mmHg) or unstable cardiovascular system
- Head or face trauma
- Lack of compliance
- Pneumothorax

- Bronchopleural fistula
- Acute asthma and bronchospasm.

If a patient has excess secretions, intermittent CPAP should be considered as this allows the patient to expectorate.

Table 2.2: Complications of non-invasive continuous positive airways pressure (CPAP)

Complication	Cause
Gastric distension and vomiting	Patient swallowing large amounts of air
Hypotension	Increased intrathoracic pressure and decreased venous return
Patient intolerance	CPAP may feel unpleasant and makes it more difficult for patient to breathe. Can feel claustrophobic
Pressure sores on nose	Mask fits very tightly with elastic straps and ears
Aspiration	Patient may vomit and be unable to remove the mask
Dry mouth/dehydration	High flow of oxygen; strict fluid balance chart needs to be maintained
Dry eyes, corneal and retinal damage	Gases escaping from the top of the mask, and blowing into the eyes

Monitoring and observations when patient is receiving non-invasive CPAP

- Pre-CPAP observations
- Monitor SpO_2 continuously
- Monitor blood pressure and pulse at least hourly
- Monitor respiratory rate at least hourly
- Perform blood gas analysis before commencing treatment, 30 minutes after start of treatment and as necessary
- Monitor conscious level by using the Glasgow coma score or a similar tool
- Perform hourly checks on the flow of gas into the system, and the temperature and water level of the humidifier
- Assess pressure areas on face/ears and head/mask fitment

- Maintain a record of CPAP observations and safety checks. This document contains an audit chart to facilitate this
- Fluid balance chart.

When the patient's condition improves, he/she can be weaned from CPAP by reducing the oxygen and PEEP delivered (*Appendix 3*).

Non-invasive ventilation

Non-invasive ventilation (NIV) is the application of positive pressure ventilation via a face or nasal mask. It allows the patient the benefits of supportive ventilation without the risks associated with endotracheal intubation. Since publication of the British Thoracic Society guidelines in 2002 there has been an increase in the number of ward areas that will accept patients for this type of support. Patients can receive NIV on general ward areas, where nurses, physiotherapists or technicians generally deliver this care. See Woodrow (2003a, b) for further information.

Tracheostomy

Tracheostomy is becoming common in acute ward areas and is no longer only seen within critical care or specialist surgical areas. General nurses therefore need to have a basic understanding of tracheostomy management and the possible complications. In this section, we consider the basics of tracheostomy care.

A tracheostomy is a surgical opening in the anterior wall of the trachea. It is generally performed to facilitate ventilation, and a tracheostomy tube is inserted (*Figure 2.12*) to

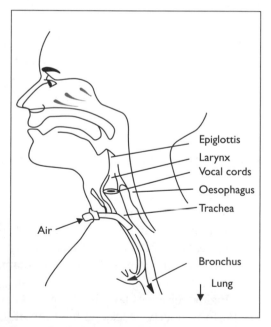

Figure 2.12: Anatomy and placement of a tracheostomy tube

keep the stoma open. This tube can be removed for cleaning. The patient's breath enters the trachea directly and then the lungs, as an alternative to breathing in and out through the nose and mouth. This reduces the dead space and makes the work of breathing easier.

Indications for a tracheostomy

Within a critical care setting a tracheostomy is often performed in patients who are likely to require prolonged and assisted ventilation. The formation of a tracheostomy allows the patient to be weaned from sedation and is more comfortable for the patient than an endotracheal tube. In patients with head injury leading to upper airway obstruction, congenital malformation or upper airway inflammation, a tracheostomy may be performed to facilitate spontaneous breathing and maintain an adequate airway.

In patients with pneumonia, a tracheostomy may be used to facilitate tracheal suction and prevent the build-up of secretions that may lead to hypoxia and hypercapnia when the patient returns to a general ward area. In patients with chronic diseases who develop respiratory insufficiency as a result of pulmonary, cardiovascular or muscular disease, and those with pharyngeal or laryngeal paralysis due to motor neurone disease, a tracheostomy may be performed to reduce the work of breathing and extend life expectancy.

Complications of a tracheostomy

- Pneumothorax
- Emphysema
- Tube displacement
- Swallowing dysfunction
- Vocal cord immobility
- Bleeding
- Infection
- Tracheoesophageal fistula
- Tracheal stenosis.

Care of a tracheostomy

Nursing priorities when caring for a patient within a general ward area who has a tracheostomy in situ should always include having the skills to remove, clean and change an inner tube in order to reduce the risk of blockage and subsequent respiratory arrest. If the patient's tracheostomy tube does not have a removable inner tube, the nurse should obtain advice from the critical care team or other appropriate source. The nurse should also:

- Encourage deep breathing to ensure that the lung bases are expanded.
- Suction only as needed. Extra caution is required in patients with a tracheostomy in situ for <72 hours as frequent suctioning may increase bleeding.
- Be able to provide humidified oxygen if necessary to loosen secretions.
- Clean the stoma and inner cannula at least 4 hourly, and change dressing every 8–12 hours.
- Change soiled tracheostomy ties as needed, but at least once a day.
- In the unlikely event that a cuff is still inflated in the ward patient, maintain minimal occlusive volume pressure in the tracheostomy cuff. Consult the product information about maximal cuff pressure.
- Keep an emergency replacement tracheostomy of the same size and next smaller size tube at the bedside.
- Consider contacting the speech and language team to teach effective communication methods, and ensure that all care providers are informed of the communication method and the patient's special communication needs.
- Provide stoma care. In order to complete tracheostomy care, the following equipment is required:
  - Dressing trolley
  - Dressing pack
  - Tracheostomy dressing
  - Sterile saline
  - Tracheostomy tapes
  - Barrier solution if necessary.

The patient should be informed of the intended procedure. The stoma should be cleaned with sterile solution using a sterile technique. If the skin around the stoma site is red or inflamed, frequent care is indicated; a barrier solution could also be considered and applied. The tissue viability nurse will be able to assess the patient and provide appropriate advice on the most appropriate barrier creams and solutions.

A pre-cut dressing needs to be placed around the tracheostomy tube to aid patient comfort and reduce tissue breakdown. The tracheostomy tapes should be changed at least daily. This procedure requires two members of staff: one to hold the tube in place to ensure that it does not become dislodged while the other changes the tapes. Tracheostomy stoma care should be completed at least once a day, although the actual frequency will depend on the individual patient: if a patient has excessive secretions, he/she should be assessed and care completed accordingly.

Changing the inner tube

The inner tube should be checked at least four hourly for patency, unless otherwise indicated. If the inner cannula is reusable, it can be removed and rinsed in sterile water at least four hourly. If it is disposable, it can be removed and checked at least four hourly, and then replaced by a new tube if it is dirty. Check what type of tube is being used locally and ensure that you are familiar with it.

The nurse should observe the tube to ascertain whether it is clean, and whether the secretions are thick and at risk of causing tube blockage, and then document the findings *(Table 2.3)*. The type of secretions that are removed when suctioned, and whether the patient coughs, should also be observed and documented.

Additional care needs in patients with long-term tracheostomies

- Continue the interventions outlined above as needed.
- Arrange for total change of tracheostomy as needed, but at least every four weeks for adults. Check the manufacturer's instructions for maximum time that the tube can remain in situ.
- Record type, size, and manufacturer of the tracheostomy tube, and document the date of insertion and last change.

Equipment to be kept by the bed of a patient with a tracheostomy:

- Tracheal dilators
- Two spare tracheostomy tubes (same size and a size smaller)
- 10ml syringe
- Spare inner tube
- Inner tube brush
- Working suction module and correct size suction catheters
- Apron
- Gloves
- Suction documentation chart.

Emergency equipment for airway management should be available on the ward but does not need to be kept at the bedside.

Table 2.3: Example of a tracheostomy care record

Date Time	%O$_2$	Resp rate	SpO$_2$	Humidification: water level checked	Suction carried out	No - Why not Yes - amount, type, colour	Inner tube cleaned	Signature
2/3/03 14.20	40%	18	96%	Bottle changed	No	Reviewed by physio. Chest clear - last suction 1 hour ago	Yes - sticky	*J. Smith*

Suctioning

Suctioning of the trachea and oropharynx is an important skill. Patients who are unable to clear their secretions will have worse gas exchange and be at greater risk of deterioration. Suction can be performed via a tracheostomy, a nasopharangeal airway into the trachea, or a Yankauer sucker into the oropharageal space. In this section we consider suctioning via a tracheostomy, as it is the method most commonly used in general ward areas. The principles are the same for any suctioning method. You should ensure that you are familiar with the equipment in your area.

Tracheal suctioning via a tracheostomy tube

Suctioning is carried out on all patients with a tracheostomy, and is an essential aspect of caring for a patient with a tracheostomy. The aim of tracheostomy suctioning is to maintain a patent airway and remove secretions.

Suctioning should not be carried out as a routine procedure; however, ensuring that a tracheostomy remains patent should be a regular action. Removing the inner tube and cleaning it with sterile water at least 4 hourly will ensure that the lumen remains clear.

Patient assessment before suctioning

- What is the respiratory rate and pattern of breathing?
- Can you hear audible rattling or bubbling of secretions?
- Are breathing sounds noisy?
- What colour is the skin?
- Are there signs of hypoxia (eg. fall in SpO_2 or cyanosis)?
- Has the patient been coughing and can you see visible amounts of secretions inside the tracheostomy tube?
- If there has been an increase in coughing, has there been effective airway clearance?

Suctioning procedure

- Assess patient for the need to suction.
- Explain the procedure to the patient, and what he/she might feel.
- Ensure that a non-fenestrated inner tube is in place.

- Turn on the suction pressure gauge; 100–120mmhg (14–16kPa) in adults is suggested (Regan, 1988; Buglass, 1999; Docherty, 2001).
- Put on gloves.
- Attach suction catheter to suction tubing. Ensure that suction catheter diameter is half the diameter of the tracheostomy tube (see *Table 2.4*).
- Ask patient to take some deep breaths.
- Observe patient at all times during the procedure.
- Insert the suction catheter into the tracheostomy tube until it reaches just beyond the end of the tube.
- Apply suction pressure by covering the hole with your finger.
- Slowly withdraw the catheter, without rotation and within 10 seconds.
- Dispose of the suction catheter, following infection control procedures.
- Reassess and repeat as necessary

Potential complications of suctioning

- Hypoxia: Suction-induced hypoxia may occur during tracheal suctioning because oxygen as well as the secretions are removed. The lower the initial SpO_2 saturation the greater the decrease in SpO_2 saturation during suctioning (Skelley *et al*, 1980). In order to prevent this complication, the patient may be asked to take some deep breaths pre- and post-suction. In patients who already have low oxygenation, suctioning time should be kept to a minimum, but should still be performed if indicated.

- Cardiac arrhythmias: The vagal nerve supplies the trachea and also the heart. On suctioning, the nerve is stimulated by the catheter touching the tracheal mucosa; this may cause cardiac arrhythmias, which are usually seen as bradycardia. There is therefore a risk of hypotension and loss of cardiac output.

- Atelectasis (collapse of the alveoli): Atelectasis may be worsened by the prolonged suctioning of air from the respiratory tract, which in turn reduces the volume of air in the alveoli.

- Trauma and bleeding: The use of high suction pressures can damage the mucous membranes. Poor humidification can also lead to drying of the mucous membranes, rendering them more susceptible to trauma from the suction catheter.

- Infection: Bacteria can be introduced as a result of poor suction technique; asepsis should therefore be maintained when suctioning.

■ Obstruction: This tends to occur when secretions block the tube. It has been identified as a spontaneous event; however, research suggests that blockage may occur through lack of humidification and lack of suction, or lack of checking and cleaning the inner tube (Corbridge, 1998). Worst scenario is a respiratory arrest.

■ Elevation of intracranial pressure: When nursing a patient with an acute head injury, cerebrovascular accident or subarachnoid haemorrhage, the nurse should be aware that suctioning will raise intracranial pressure by making the patient cough, which in turn may exacerbate the cerebral oedema.

Common questions when suctioning

Which size suction catheter should I use?

Suction catheters are available in a variety of sizes, and you need to be familiar with what is available locally. They need to have a port on the side to allow pressure to be applied intermittently, and several holes at the tip to collect secretions. The consensus in the literature is that the diameter of the suction catheter should be half the diameter of the tracheostomy tube (DeCarle, 1985). To find the size of suction catheter needed, multiply the tracheostomy size by two and then subtract two. For example, a size six tracheostomy tube would require a suction catheter size (6 x 2) – 2, which equals 10. *Table 2.4* summarises the suction catheter sizes required for various tracheostomy tube sizes.

What suction pressure should I use?

Suctioning is the drawing of air out of a space to create a vacuum, which will then suck in surrounding liquids (Griggs, 1999), ie. secretions in tracheostomy suctioning.

Table 2.4: Tracheostomy tube and suction catheter sizes

Tracheostomy tube size	Suction catheter size
10	18
9	16
8	14
7	12
6	10

Within all hospital settings, suction apparatus have a pressure control dial. If the pressure is set too low, suctioning the patient's airway will be ineffective and cause the patient undue distress. If the pressure is set too high, the suction catheter can adhere to the tracheal wall, damaging the tracheal mucosa and causing atelectasis. Serra *et al* (2000) and Regan (1988) support the view that an increased pressure will lead to mucosal damage, and is not necessarily more effective or efficient in the removal of secretions. Research has identified a variety of ideal pressure settings for adult suctioning (Regan, 1988; Odell *et al*, 1993; Griggs, 1999; Day, 2000). From this research it would seem that a setting between 16kPa and 20kPa should be adopted.

The setting on the suction system should always be checked before commencing tracheal suctioning, and the lowest amount of pressure needed to remove the secretions should be used. Suction is applied by covering the air port at the top of the catheter with a thumb as the catheter is removed; the reason for doing it this way is that damage would be caused to the mucous membranes if suction were applied as the catheter was inserted.

Should I rotate the catheter during suctioning?

Within the medical and surgical wards, multi-eyed catheters are now available. Formerly, single-eyed catheters were in use and practice included rotation on removal. This is old practice, and is no longer recommended. The multi-eyed catheter has holes around the catheter, and is therefore able to draw in secretions without rotation.

How far should I insert the catheter?

This varies according to the patient's status. If a patient is awake and able to cough secretions to the end of the tracheostomy tube, the suction catheter need only be inserted to the end of the tube. However, patients with an impaired cough reflex due to their illness may have an accumulation of secretions in the lower respiratory tract. In the case of limited or no cough reflex, the catheter is inserted until resistance is felt and then withdrawn slightly, before suction and withdrawal. The point of resistance occurs at the carina – the point where the trachea divides into two bronchi.

How long can I take to suction?

The full procedure from insertion of the catheter to removal of the catheter should take no longer than fifteen seconds. While withdrawing the catheter, intermittent suction is applied – this should be done for no longer than ten seconds before releasing and reapplying until the catheter is fully removed (Day *et al*, 2002).

Key learning points for *Chapter 2*

- Always record respiratory rate.
- The ability to cough is important: if the patient cannot cough then a physiotherapist should be asked to assess the patient and help plan care to ensure that coughing is possible.
- Remember that oxygen saturation has limitations and only measures the saturation of available haemoglobin: it does not indicate carbon dioxide levels.
- Gas exchange takes place in the alveoli; if they are full of secretions or fluid, gas exchange will be reduced.
- Increasing functional residual capacity (FRC) will increase the patient's ability for gas exchange. The application of continuous positive airways pressure (CPAP) will increase FRC.
- The diaphragm is the biggest respiratory muscle. If its ability to function is reduced because of pain, abdominal distension, abdominal surgery or neurological damage, the risk of respiratory failure is increased (summarised in *Appendix 4*).
- Chemoreceptors in the carotid bodies and aortic arch respond to changes in carbon dioxide level, and send messages to the respiratory centre in the brain to change the rate of respiration.
- Atmospheric air contains 21% oxygen.
- Prevention of respiratory failure and improvement in respiratory function can be achieved by basic measures such as sitting the patient up, encouraging coughing, ensuring adequate hydration and good pain relief.
- Tracheostomies need regular observation to ensure that secretions do not block the tube. Ensure that you are competent to check an inner tube.
- Chest tubes and drainage systems must be kept patent. The underwater seal must be maintained and bottles kept upright.

Revision questions – respiratory care

1. Peter Smith, a 48-year-old taxi driver, is admitted with shortness of breath. He has a respiratory rate of 28 breaths/min and his O_2 saturation is 92% on air. His blood pressure is 140/80mmHg and heart rate is 74 beats/min. He has a temperature of 37.8°C. Peter smokes twenty cigarettes a day. He has a productive cough and his sputum is green.

What are your priorities in his care?

2. Mary Jones is a 72-year-old woman who had a total abdominal hysterectomy four days ago. This morning she feels short of breath and her observations are:

- Blood pressure 160/90mmHg
- Heart rate 95 beats/min
- Respiratory rate 30 breaths/min
- Temperature 38°C
- SpO_2 88% on air

What are your concerns in this woman, and what is the possible diagnosis? What are your actions?

Answers on page 196

References

British Thoracic Society (2002) Non-invasive ventilation in acute respiratory failure. *Thorax* **57**(3): 192–211

Buglass E (1999) Tracheostomy care: tracheal suctioning and humidification. *British Journal of Nursing* **8**(8): 500–04

Casey D (1989) Open airways. *Nursing Standard* **3**(22): 19–20

Corbridge R (1998) *Essential ENT Practice: A clinical text*. Arnold, London: 40–60

Day T (2000) Tracheal suctioning: when, why and how. *Nursing Times* **96**(20): 13–15

Day T, Farnell S, Wilson-Barnett J (2002) Suctioning: a review of current research recommendations. *Intensive and Critical Care Nursing* **18**(2): 79–89

DeCarle B (1985) Tracheostomy care. *Nursing Times* **81**(40): 50–4

Docherty B (2001) Tracheostomy care. Clinical Practice Review. *Professional Nurse* **16**(8): 1272

Griggs A (1999) Tracheostomy: suctioning and humidification. *Emergency Nurse* **6**(9): 33–40

Odell A, Allder A, Bayne R *et al* (1993) Endotracheal suction for adult non-head injured patients. *Intensive Critical Care Nursing* **9**: 274–78

Regan M (1988) Tracheal mucosal injury: the nurse's role. *Nursing* **3**(29): 1064–66

Serra A (2000) Tracheostomy care. *Nursing Standard* **14**(42): 45–52

Skelley BF, Deeren SM, Powaser MM (1980) The effectiveness of two preoxygenation methods to prevent endotracheal suction-induced hypoxemia. *Heart and Lung* **9**(2) 316–23

Woodrow P (2003a) Using non-invasive ventilation in acute wards. Part 1. *Nursing Standard* **18**(1): 39–44

Woodrow P (2003b) Using non-invasive ventilation in acute wards. Part 2. *Nursing Standard* **18**(2): 41–4

Woodrow P (2004) Arterial blood gas analysis. *Nursing Standard* **18**(21): 45–52

CHAPTER 3

Cardiovascular care

P Pratt

Assessment and observations

History

When assessing a patient for cardiovascular problems, the history is important. The nurse needs to ask the following questions:

- Has the patient got or had any chest pain?
- What was the pain like – was it stabbing, crushing, sharp, continuous, etc.?
- Has the patient had any dizziness, blackouts or fainting episodes?
- Does the patient have a cardiac history (previous myocardial infarction, angina or hypertension)?
- Is the patient on any cardiac medication?
- Is there a family history of cardiac disease?

Assessment

You need to assess the patient's current cardiovascular status. This includes:

- Is the patient responding to you?
- Are the observations normal or abnormal?
- Is the patient clammy or sweaty?
- Does the patient currently have any chest pain?
- Does the patient feel dizzy?
- Does the patient have a good colour?

Observations

Blood pressure

Blood pressure is the pressure exerted against the blood vessel walls; each type of blood vessel has a different normal pressure. When we talk clinically on an acute ward about blood pressure, we are generally referring to arterial blood pressure and this is what we measure. This is an important pressure, as it must be maintained to ensure that blood flow to the vital organs is adequate. On general wards, blood pressure is often recorded by automatic machines; however, when a patient has a very low blood pressure it is important for the nurse to be able to measure blood pressure manually using a sphygmomanometer, as automatic blood pressure measuring equipment may be inaccurate in this situation.

Simple measures to ensure accurate measurement of blood pressure include:

- Use a cuff of the correct size
- Ensure that the arm is supported and at heart level
- Avoid recording the blood pressure after a meal
- Be aware of the effect of pain or anxiety on the recording
- Ensure that the patient is in a comfortable position
- Try to use the same arm for each recording.

If a reading does not seem to fit the clinical picture of the patient, check the reading again.

Central venous pressure

Central venous pressure (CVP) is measured in the large veins before they enter the heart. It gives an indication of fluid status and cardiac failure. Further information on reading a CVP will be given later.

Heart rate and rhythm

The nurse should always take a pulse by feeling the patient's radial artery, and not by recording it from the automatic reading devices used in most acute wards. Feeling the pulse manually will enable more information to be gained about the patient's cardiac output, such as:

- Is the heart rate regular?
- Is it thready and weak?
- Is it bounding?
- Is the patient cold and clammy?

Cardiac rhythm is important in the acutely ill adult and needs careful interpretation. It may be necessary to monitor cardiac rhythm continuously in acutely ill adults, as these patients are at increased risk of cardiovascular problems. By monitoring cardiac rhythm, the nurse is able to assess deviations from normal, and respond to abnormal rhythms before cardiovascular function becomes compromised. Some patients may have asymptomatic rhythm changes, while others may be in a collapsed state or in cardiac arrest. The ward nurse needs to be able to identify normal sinus rhythm and some common general arrhythmias. This chapter will cover basic cardiac monitoring only – not 12-lead electrocardiogram (ECG) interpretations.

The electrocardiogram

The electrical impulses that produce the cardiac muscle contraction can be recorded from electrodes placed on the body surface. The graphic recording (trace) obtained is termed the ECG.

An ECG may be obtained with 12 separate leads (views) from 10 electrodes attached to the patient. The 12-lead ECG is used in the diagnosis of arrhythmias and acute coronary syndromes. In this book, we will consider only the single-lead ECG, ie. basic cardiac monitoring, which may be carried out in general ward areas. Readers who wish to explore this area further should consult the bibliography.

It is important to note that single-lead monitoring and 12-lead ECG monitoring refer to different views of the heart. A graphic representation of the measurement of impulses passing towards or away from 12 different points (leads) in the heart can seen on paper or on a cardiac monitor screen. To obtain a single-lead view, three electrodes are connected to the patient as shown in *Figure 3.1*. When the chest electrodes and cables are connected in this way, the monitor needs to be configured to view 'lead II'; the trace shown in *Figure 3.2* should be seen. *Figure 3.3* shows the times of the different phases of the normal ECG during one contraction and relaxation of the heart.

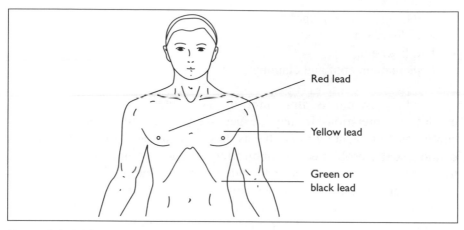

Figure 3.1: ECG lead placement for basic cardiac monitoring

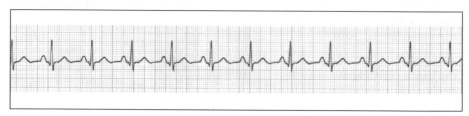

Figure 3.2: Normal ECG monitoring trace

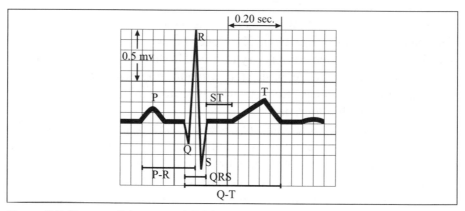

Figure 3.3: Phases of the normal ECG

Interpreting an ECG – common rules

Before attempting to interpret any cardiac rhythm, always check your patient first. Is there a pulse, is the patient conscious and are any of his/her vital organs compromised (ie. are blood pressure and/or conscious level affected by the change in cardiac rhythm)? Once you have assessed your patient, and called for help if necessary, you can then follow a series of questions to identify the rhythm:

- Can P waves be seen? Are they regular?
- Is there a P wave before every QRS complex?
- Is the space between the P wave and QRS complex equivalent to two small squares?
- Is the PR interval longer than five small squares?
- Is the QRS complex positive?
- Is the QRS complex greater than three small squares?
- Are the QRS complexes regular?

Anatomy and physiology

Basic anatomy

The heart lies in the mediastinum and consists of four chambers: right atrium, left atrium, right ventricle and left ventricle *(Figure 3.4)*. Its function is to act as a pump, pushing oxygenated blood to the body and vital organs and deoxygenated blood to the lungs.

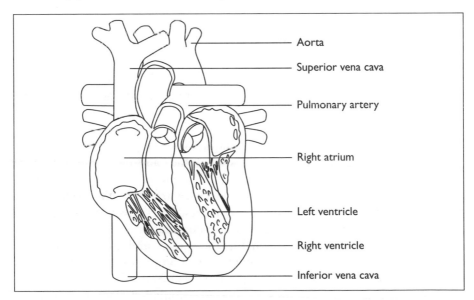

Figure 3.4: Basic anatomy of the heart

Cardiac muscle cells make up the myocardium, which is lined with endocardium on the inside and enclosed by epicardium on the outside. Cardiac muscle is striated and the myofibrils contain actin and myosin. Between each cell there are intercalated discs, which have low resistance to the passage of electrical impulses, and so allow action potentials to travel along the fibres quite easily.

Mechanics of the heart

Cardiac output is the amount of blood pumped from the left ventricle into the aorta each minute. Cardiac output is determined by the amount of blood pumped by the left ventricle during each beat and the number of beats per minute. The amount of blood moved during each beat is the stroke volume. In an adult at rest, the stroke volume is about 70ml.

Cardiac output	=	Stroke volume x beats per minute
	=	70ml x 75 beats per minute
	=	5250ml per minute

Physiology

Chemical control of the heart

Compensatory mechanisms affecting heart rate are triggered if cardiac output falls too low to maintain adequate organ perfusion. A very low cardiac output puts the patient at considerable risk. Damage to the myocardium or blood loss can cause a fall in cardiac output. The body tries to compensate by increasing the heart rate. When stimulated, the cardio-acceleratory centre in the medulla oblongata of the brain sends impulses, via the sympathetic nerves, to the sinoatrial (SA) node and atrioventricular (AV) node, which result in the release of norepinephrine (noradrenaline); this is detected by the SA and AV nodes, leading to an increase in heart rate.

The medulla oblongata also contains the cardio-inhibitory centre. When stimulated, the cardio-inhibitory centre sends impulses down the vagus nerve to the SA and AV nodes, causing the release of acetylcholine, which slows the heart rate. Both centres respond to stimulation from baroreceptors to cause a change in heart rate and cardiac output.

Baroreceptors (also called pressoreceptors) located in the carotid arteries and aortic arch are nerve endings that detect the amount of stretch generated in these vessels. They respond to changes in blood pressure and have reflex actions. The carotid and aortic reflexes work in the same way. They are concerned with maintaining normal blood pressure in the brain and other vital organs. When the baroreceptors detect stretching, they send impulses via the glossopharyneal nerve to the brain to inhibit the cardio-acceleratory centre, which results in a reduction in heart rate and strength of contractions and hence a lowering of blood pressure. If the baroreceptors detect a decrease in pressure, the cardio-inhibitory centre is inhibited, leading to an increase in heart rate and strength of contractions, and hence a rise in blood pressure.

Chemicals in the bloodstream can also affect the heart rate. Electrolyte abnormalities can affect heart rate and rhythm. Potassium is thought to effect the generation of nerve impulses, and sodium excess to effect muscular contraction.

Effect of temperature

A rise in body temperature increases the rate of production of impulses from the AV node, thereby increasing the heart rate. If body temperature falls, the release of impulses from the AV node is slowed and thus heart rate decreases.

Electrical control of the heart

In normal resting adults, cardiac muscle tissue relaxes and contracts around 70 times a minute. This means that the cells have a constant need for oxygen delivery and carbon dioxide removal. Cardiac muscle contracts without an extrinsic stimulus, as the cells have automaticity. However, an extrinsic stimulus can affect the rate of depolarisation. Cardiac muscle cells also differ from other muscle tissue in that they have a longer period of relaxation owing to the length of time over which repolarisation occurs. This allows the heart chamber to fill before contraction occurs again. Following the action potential there is a period during which the cardiac muscle does not respond, ensuring that enough time is allowed for relaxation of the muscle and, in the case of the myocardium, filling of the heart chambers.

Resting potential

A cell at rest has a resting membrane potential, which is dependent on the permeability of the cell membrane to potassium ions (K+) and sodium ions (Na+), and to the concentrations of these two electrolytes both inside and outside the cell. At rest the cell membrane is more permeable to K+ than Na+; hence K+ moves out of the cell, making the inside of the cell more negative with respect to the outside. When the threshold potential is reached, permeability to Na+ increases and Na+ moves into the cell, making the inside of the cell less negative than the outside.

This movement of Na+ and K+ and the rapid reversal of positive and negative charges inside the cell constitutes the action potential. In a cardiac muscle cell, depolarisation lasts for around 0.15–0.3 seconds, allowing the impulse to be transferred across all the cardiac cells, and making the heart an efficient pump.

Starling's Law states that the force of contraction of cardiac muscle is proportional to the stretched length of the muscle fibre. The length of the fibres and amount of stretch that occurs are influenced by the amount of blood in the heart chambers before contraction. It is important that the heart has enough time to fill with blood and hence stretch the heart chamber so that it can then eject the blood into the body via the aorta. This is why we need to ensure that the patient is not hypovolaemic or overloaded. The patient's cardiovascular system needs to be adequately 'filled', and for this we can use a central venous pressure (CVP) line.

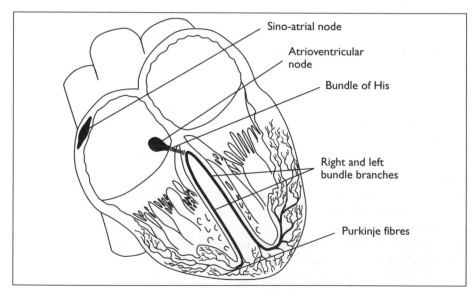

Figure 3.5: Conduction pathways of the heart

Conduction pathways of the heart

We have considered how the muscle fibres are stimulated to contract and relax. This needs to occur in a coordinated manner, hence the heart has a specific pathway that leads to the stimulation of an action potential across the myocardium. This includes the SA node, the AV node, the AV bundle (bundle of His) and the right and left bundle branches *(Figure 3.5)*.

Additional learning point

Ectopic beats: The SA node is the heart's pacemaker, but all cardiac cells have the ability to contract without any extrinsic stimulus, therefore if an impulse is generated by a cell outside the normal path it may be seen on the ECG as an ectopic beat. Ectopic beats can be caused by ischaemia, hypoxia, electrolyte disorders, stress, caffeine and nicotine.

Cardiovascular diseases

Angina pectoris

Angina is defined as cardiac chest pain due to ischaemia of the myocardium brought on by exercise and relieved by rest or nitrates.

Risk factors

*   Smoking
*   Hypertension
*   Increasing age
*   Gender
*   Family history
*   Obesity
*   Diabetes
*   Stress
*   Lack of exercise

Signs and symptoms

- Chest pain on exertion
- Pain radiating into the arm and neck
- Pain felt as a tight band around the chest
- Shortness of breath

Key problems

Patients with angina have an increased risk of myocardial infarction and are also at risk of life-threatening arrhythmias. The nurse must treat any chest pain in a timely manner and ensure that the patient is supported, in order to alleviate any increased anxiety.

Acute coronary syndromes

Acute coronary syndromes represent myocardial ischaemia, which causes the patient to present with chest pain that is not relieved by rest or nitrates and is often associated with ECG changes. Acute coronary syndromes include ST elevation MI (STEMI), non-ST elevation MI (non-STEMI) and unstable angina.

Risk factors

- Smoking
- Hypertension
- Hypercholesterolaemia
- History of coronary artery disease
- Stress
- Increasing age
- Gender
- Family history
- Obesity
- Diabetes
- Lack of exercise

Signs and symptoms

- Central crushing chest pain not relieved by rest or nitrates
- Sweating and feeling of impending doom

- Possible ECG changes
- Arrhythmias
- Shortness of breath
- Hypotension
- Tachycardia
- Cardiac arrest

Key problems

The patient will be very anxious, and treatments must be delivered in a calm, reassuring manner. Pain relief should be given and its effectiveness monitored; further pain relief should be given if needed. Close monitoring and observation are necessary to ensure early recognition of arrhythmia and cardiac failure.

Cardiac failure

Cardiac failure is defined as inadequate blood pressure and cardiac output to meet basic body requirements. Cardiac failure can be left- or right-sided only, and these may occur independently or jointly (Swanton, 1998).

Risks

Any problem – direct or indirect – that reduces cardiac output will contribute to cardiac failure. Some contributing factors are:

- Myocardial infarction
- Sepsis
- Shock
- Haemorrhage
- Trauma
- Arrhythmias
- Hypertension.

Signs and symptoms

- Fall in blood pressure
- Changes in conscious level

- Reduction in urine output
- Increase in heart rate
- Pulmonary oedema
- Fatigue
- Shortness of breath – laying flat, on exertion or at rest
- Peripheral oedema

Key problems

If the patient is unable to maintain an adequate cardiac output, other body systems will start to fail. The nurse's role is to optimise blood pressure, and in turn cardiac function, by the administration and monitoring of fluids, drugs and oxygen. The cause of the cardiac failure needs to be established so that corrective treatment can be given (eg. if the cause is arrhythmia, then anti-arrhythmic drugs will need to be administered).

Close observation and reporting of abnormal blood pressure and early intervention are the nurse's primary objectives.

Shock

Shock is defined as the failure of cardiac output and tissue oxygenation to meet the needs of the vital organs. There are several types of shock, all of which are named according to their primary cause. They are:

- Cardiogenic shock
- Hypovolaemic shock
- Septic shock
- Anaphylactic shock
- Neurogenic shock

Shock progresses in three stages: stage 1 (compensated), stage 2 (decompensated) and stage 3 (irreversible). Within the ward setting it is important for the nurse to be able to identify stage 1 shock and report the findings to medical staff so that action can be taken to slow or prevent progression.

- Stage 1 shock – Compensated: At this point the normal physiological responses of the body are compensating for early signs of shock in order to maintain tissue perfusion and oxygenation. This will include changes in heart rate, urine output and perfusion of vital organs. It is important to note that the blood pressure will be normal. The nurse must consider the patient's likely risk factors and the possible cause of shock by observing current signs and symptoms (eg. if the patient has just had surgery, he/she may be bleeding, or if the patient has an infection, he/she could be developing septic shock).

- Stage 2 shock – Decompensated: When the body systems are no longer able to compensate and physiological mechanisms are failing to preserve and maintain tissue perfusion, hypoxia will start to increase. At this point, blood pressure will start to fall. The patient may become confused or complain of chest pain as vital organs are deprived of oxygen. This stage is still reversible, but actions must be taken quickly and the underlying cause must be identified and treated.

- Stage 3 – Irreversible: At this point the body systems are struggling to cope, and damage to vital organs has occurred. If untreated, stage 3 shock will lead to death. It cannot be stressed enough that the entire aim is to prevent stage 3 shock.

Additional learning point

It is important that shock is identified as early as possible to prevent it progressing to stage 3.

Risk factors

There are many risk factors for shock, and these are often related to the type of shock. The risk factors for each type of shock are summarised below. Appendix 5 shows a flow diagram to assist in assessing the patient for septic shock.

Septic shock

- Wound infections
- Cross-infection
- Reduced immunity
- Intravenous lines
- Parenteral nutrition
- Urinary catheter

Hypovolaemic shock

- Bleeding
- Fluid loss

Cardiogenic shock

- Myocardial infarction
- Arrhythmias
- Fluid overload

Anaphylactic shock

- Allergies

Neurogenic shock

- Spinal cord injury

Signs and symptoms

- Tachycardia
- Oliguria
- Fall in blood pressure
- Confusion
- Vasoconstriction (occurs in hypovolaemic and cardiogenic shock)
- Vasodilatation (occurs in septic, anaphylactic and neurogenic shock)

Shock can lead to multi-organ failure due to tissue hypoxia, and this can be irreversible. Patients with severe shock will often be admitted to the intensive care unit for multisystem support, but it is necessary to consider what shock is and how to recognise the early signs so that management can be commenced. The primary physiological effect of shock, regardless of the cause, is reduced perfusion of the tissues.

Key problems

Early identification of the cause of shock must be achieved in order that it can be treated. Goal-directed therapy must be implemented in a timely manner to prevent further deterioration and organ failure. The patient who is in shock needs frequent close observation, effective intervention and accurate record keeping. He/she will often need to be moved to a higher level of care.

Cardiac arrhythmias

Arrhythmia is defined as abnormal cardiac conduction. It may affect the heart's ability to maintain adequate cardiac output.

Risk factors

- Myocardial ischaemia
- Myocardial infarction
- Electrolyte imbalance
- Shock

Signs and symptoms

- Can be asymptomatic
- Patient may be in cardiac arrest
- Chest pain
- Shortness of breath
- Dizziness
- Fainting
- Fall in blood pressure

Common cardiac arrhythmias

In this section we will consider seven common cardiac monitoring traces (*Figures 3.6–3.12*) and key points for the nurse to consider that have implications for

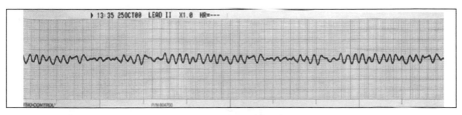

Figure 3.6: ECG monitoring trace showing ventricular fibrillation

nursing practice. The most important issue for the nurse is 'How is the patient?' Diagnosis of the arrhythmia is the next most important issue.

First, we will consider emergency arrhythmias. *Figure 3.6* shows ventricular fibrillation. Electrical activity is disorganised, hence there is no mechanical activity and no cardiac output will be felt when checking for a pulse. This is a cardiac arrest arrhythmia and needs urgent defibrillation.

Figure 3.7 shows a similar rhythm – ventricular tachycardia. This is a fast rhythm with no obvious P waves and a wide QRS complex. It originates in the ventricles and the patient is often haemodynamically compromised, with a low blood pressure, and feels dizzy or even loses consciousness. This rhythm can also be a cardiac arrest rhythm. So check your patient first. If the patient is in cardiac arrest, defibrillation will be needed. If the patient is haemodynamically compromised but has a pulse and blood pressure, urgent cardioversion is needed. Cardioversion can be achieved by electrical or pharmacological means and will be discussed later in this chapter.

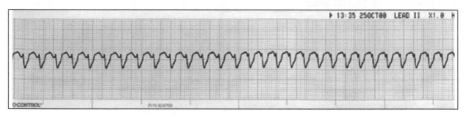

Figure 3.7: ECG monitoring trace showing ventricular tachycardia

Figure 3.8 shows a sinus bradycardia. This is defined by the presence of a normal PQRS complex, but the heart rate is slow. The rate is calculated by measuring the number of large squares between two R waves. There are 10 large squares between the two R waves in the ECG trace shown in *Figure 3.8*. So, we divide 300 (speed of the ECG machine in number of large squares per minute) by the number of large squares between the two R waves (10); this gives us a heart rate of 30 beats/min. Cardiovascular function may be compromised by this rate, and conscious level and blood pressure can be affected. The patient may feel dizzy only if he/she stands up. This arrhythmia may be a response to vomiting or receiving tracheal suction and therefore

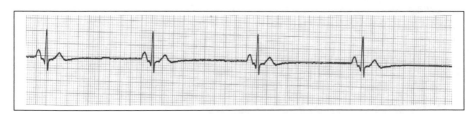

Figure 3.8: ECG monitoring trace showing sinus bradycardia

should be short-lived. If the rate does not increase and cardiovascular function becomes compromised, treatment must be given. Atropine is the drug of choice as it blocks vagal nerve activity and so reduces inhibition of the SA node, hence it should produce an increase in heart rate.

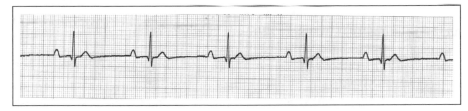

Figure 3.9: ECG monitoring trace showing first-degree heart block

When assessing bradycardias it is important to examine the ECG for heart block. This is manifest by an extension of the time taken for an impulse to pass from the atria to the ventricles. In *Figure 3.9* it can be seen that the PR interval is greater than 2 small squares, ie. longer than 0.4s; this rhythm is called first-degree heart block (block between the impulse passing from the SA node to the AV node). Most patients will be asymptomatic with this rhythm and will not require acute treatment.

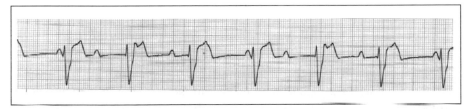

Figure 3.10: ECG monitoring trace showing complete heart block

In *Figure 3.10* the P waves and the Q waves have no association with each other, and this rhythm is termed complete heart block. Patients with this rhythm are usually compromised and generally require cardiac pacing.

In *Figure 3.11* the P waves do not always have a QRS complex following them, and some have two P waves to one QRS complex. This is a type

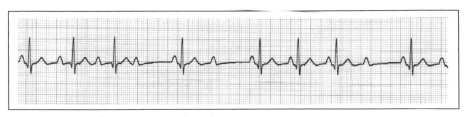

Figure 3.11: ECG monitoring trace showing type II second-degree heart block

of heart block called type II second-degree heart block. Patients with this rhythm are at risk of progressing to complete heart block, which often leads to profound bradycardia. Even the uncompromised patient with this type of heart block will require treatment, usually in the form of elective pacing.

The ECG shown in *Figure 3.12* has no P waves but a normal-looking QRS complex. This irregular pattern is atrial fibrillation (AF), ie. the atria are being stimulated by many different focal points in an erratic manner. Eventually the impulse stimulates the AV node, leading to a normal conduction across the ventricles. It is common for patients with chronic AF to receive anticoagulation, as one of the problems of AF is that the atria do not empty fully and pooled blood can form a thrombus, increasing the risk of stroke.

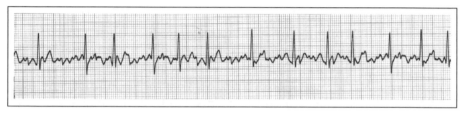

Figure 3.12: ECG monitoring trace showing atrial fibrillation

Key problems

The greatest risk for a patient who has a cardiac arrhythmia is its effect on cardiac output. The patient may feel dizzy, have 'blackouts' or, in the most serious cases, suffer full loss of cardiac output and be in cardiac arrest. If in doubt, call for senior help.

Treatments and interventions

Basics

- Oxygen: If cardiac output falls, the ability of the blood to transport oxygen is also reduced. Patients with reduced cardiac output and cardiac failure should be given oxygen as a matter of routine in order to optimise the amount of oxygen in the blood.

- Positioning: To facilitate good oxygen delivery the patient should be positioned to optimise respiratory and cardiac function. Sitting the patient in a chair with the legs raised will improve breathing, and have the least impact on cardiac output. Obviously a patient who is in shock should be nursed in bed and may need to be positioned flat with head down if blood pressure or conscious level is affected.

- Reassurance: The patient with cardiac failure will be very anxious, and may feel very breathless and fatigued; also, he/she may often have a fear of dying. Reassurance and clear explanations are important as anxiety increases the heart rate, which in turn will make the patient worse. A mild sedative may be considered in very anxious patients.

- Pain relief: If the patient has any chest pain, an analgesic can be administered. Pain issues in general are discussed in Chapter 8. Remember that analgesics can cause nausea, so an anti-emetic may also be needed.

- Fluids: Managing the patient's fluid status will optimise cardiac output if the cause of the inadequacy is hypovolaemia. The replacement fluid can be colloid (large molecules) or crystalloid (smaller molecules). If a patient has a CVP line in situ, a baseline reading should be recorded, where possible, before fluid is administered.

Fluid challenge

If a fluid challenge is requested, this indicates that a volume of fluid over and above the regular maintenance fluid is needed. The term is used loosely and no formal definition of the amount or type of fluid is available; each challenge needs to be individualised (Dellinger *et al*, 2004). The Oxford Handbook of Medicine (Longmore *et al*, 2001) suggests crystalloid fluid, usually 500–1000ml, administered over 30–60 minutes, followed by re-evaluation to check the response. However, colloid or blood may also be prescribed, in which case 300–500ml colloid over 30 minutes is suggested (Dellinger *et al*, 2004). The patient's condition and causative factors should direct the choice of fluid. The recording of baseline observations before and directly after the fluid challenge is of key importance to allow assessment of its effect and the implementation of further management.

Drugs

Thrombolytics

Thrombolytics are drugs that dissolve blood clots (thrombi). When a thrombus has formed, its dissolution is the key to optimising blood flow back to the infarcted myocardium. However, the use of thrombolytic drugs does carry risks, such as bleeding and stroke, so careful consideration of the potential benefits and risks is essential before administering these drugs. The nurse is directed to the bibliography for details on the various thrombolytics available and their contraindications. It is uncommon for staff on general wards to administer these drugs, as patients requiring them will often be transferred to a higher level of care, such as a coronary care unit or high dependency unit.

Anti-arrhythmic drugs

This group of drugs includes many different drugs that aim to stabilise the cardiac cells. In general they fall into four categories, depending on their effects on cardiac electrical activity:

- Class I drugs are sodium-channel blockers, such as lignocaine.

- Class II drugs are beta-blockers. These work by blocking beta-adrenoceptors in the heart, peripheral vascular system, bronchioles, pancreas and liver. The main actions of these drugs are to slow the heart rate and reduce contractility, so the nurse should be aware of these effects on cardiac function. As these drugs also block receptors in the bronchioles it is important for the nurse to monitor respiratory function and report any increased wheeze or shortness of breath associated with their administration.

- Class III drugs are potassium-channel blockers, such as amiodarone. This drug works by stabilising the cell membrane and converting the heart back to sinus rhythm. A common regimen is a bolus dose of amiodarone 300mg given intravenously, followed by an infusion of 900mg over 24 hours.

- Class IV drugs are calcium-channel blockers, such as verapamil.

> **Additional learning point**
> Anti-arrhythmic drugs act on the various channels that control the
> movement of sodium, potassium and calcium ions across the cardiac cell
> membrane, thereby stabilising it.

Atropine

Atropine is an anticholinergic drug that blocks vagal nerve stimulation,
thereby preventing or halting bradycardia. The usual intravenous dose is
500μg, increasing to a maximum total dose of 3mg.

Digoxin

Digoxin slows conductivity across the AV node, and thus reduces the heart
rate in atrial fibrillation. It is also a weak inotrope and therefore increases
the force of contraction of the myocardium. It is commonly given as a single
bolus of 500μg intravenously.

Diuretics

Diuretics fall into three main groups, depending on their mode of action:

- Loop diuretics, such as furosemide, act on the loop of Henle and are
  commonly used in the acutely ill patient.

- Thiazide diuretics, such as bendroflumethiazide, inhibit sodium
  absorption in the distal tubule.

- Potassium-sparing diuretics, such as amiloride, which reduce potassium
  and hydrogen ion excretion, are the weakest form of diuretics and are
  generally used in acutely ill adults.

It is important to monitor fluid balance in acutely ill patients who
are receiving diuretics, in order to determine the effect of the drugs on
urine output and other systems such as cardiovascular and respiratory
function.

Analgesics

A variety of analgesics may be used in the acutely ill adult. These are discussed in detail in *Chapter 8*; the reader should refer to *Figure 8.2*, in particular.

Advanced monitoring and support

Central venous catheters

A central venous catheter (CVC) is a line that is inserted into a major vein in the neck, groin or upper chest. The veins most commonly used are the subclavian, internal and external jugular, and the femoral veins. It is also possible to thread a central line into these larger vessels via the brachial or cephalic veins. These catheters are called peripherally inserted central catheters (PICC).

Central lines are used for:

* Administration of large volumes of fluid
* Administration of drugs
* Administration of parenteral nutrition
* Haemodynamic monitoring
* Access for renal replacement therapy.

In the general ward setting it is more common for a central line to have been inserted intraoperatively or in another treatment area, so that the patient returns to the ward with the line in situ. Occasionally a line will be inserted on a general ward and the nurse should check local policy for her role in this procedure. In this section we will consider the nurse's role in the care of the line and how to monitor CVP.

CVP measurement: Monitoring of the central line after insertion is a key nursing role. In the acutely ill patient, CVP measurement will help to guide fluid management.

CVP is a pressure in the central venous circulation that relates to volume status by allowing estimation of fluid volume, vascular tone and right heart function. Normal CVP is 3–8mmHg (5–13cmH$_2$O). On a general ward, CVP is commonly measured via a water manometer rather than a pressure transducer, which is used in most critical care areas. It is important to remember that CVP readings indicate a trend, and caution should be taken with single readings. CVP measurements must also be read in conjunction with any other observations being recorded, eg. heart rate, blood pressure, urine output and respiratory rate.

How to read a water manometer:

1. Set up a reading system by attaching the central venous line, via the distal port, to a manometer tubing set and then to a bag of fluid, usually normal saline, as shown in *Figure 3.13*.

2. Fill the water column (A), which lays alongside the measuring device, with normal saline (B) by turning the three-way tap off to the patient line, thereby opening the line between the fluid and water column.

3. When the column is filled, move the zero point on the measuring device so that it is positioned level with the patient's right atrium.

4. Close off the three-way tap from the saline bag, and open the tap between the measuring column and the patient (C). The level of fluid should then fall to a stable height on the measuring column. The position at which the column becomes stable is the CVP reading. A 'swing' in the water level may be seen, owing to the slight movement of the water column with respiration.

5. Finally, turn the three-way tap so that normal saline flows to the patient from the reservoir bag, keeping the line patent. The reservoir bag usually has a volume of 500ml and will run over approximately 24 hours.

Drug administration via a central line: Some drugs can only be given via a large vein, owing to the toxicity of the drugs and the damage they may cause to smaller vessels. Also, giving a drug via a central line will ensure that its action is optimised as soon as possible, as it is delivered directly into the central circulation. However, this also means that any adverse reaction will occur sooner and may be more severe.

When giving drugs via a central venous line the

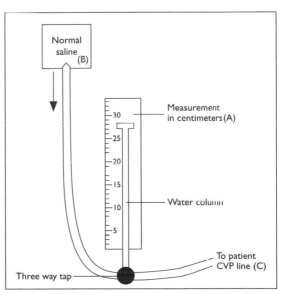

Figure 3.13: Water manometer set-up for measuring central venous pressure

nurse should ensure that aseptic technique is adhered to, as the line has the potential to become infected, with severe consequences. The line should be flushed before and after giving drugs so that precipitation and mixing of the drugs does not occur in the line.

Risks of central venous line use: Caution should be taken with central venous lines, as there are several risks associated with their use. The benefits of using the line should outweigh the possible risks and complications. The patient should also give informed consent where possible.

The patient should be observed for possible complications. After a central venous line has been inserted, its position should be confirmed by X-ray before it is used by the nurse. Potential complications include:

- Air embolism
- Thrombus formation
- Infection at the insertion site
- Line infection
- Pneumothorax
- Haematoma
- Embolism
- Arrhythmias due to line position
- Haemorrhage
- Risks associated with disconnection.

The line should be removed as soon as it is no longer necessary, in order to avoid undue risks.

Cardioversion

Cardioversion may be performed by pharmacological or electrical means. We have considered the drugs that may be used to control heart rhythm, and here we discuss the use of an electrical current delivered to the myocardium to revert an arrhythmia to sinus rhythm.

The patient will be sedated or anaesthetised, and will have a defibrillator placed on his/her chest. The position of the paddles and the machine will be the same as those used for defibrillation in a cardiac arrest. The defibrillator must be synchronised with the patient's heart rhythm so that the shock is discharged on the R wave to reduce the risk of ventricular fibrillation. This treatment is generally only given in a coronary care unit or critical care unit.

Cardiac pacing

If the heart rate is too slow to maintain an adequate cardiac output and blood pressure, it may be necessary to stimulate the heart with an electric current. This current is delivered at a set rate in order to trigger contraction and generate cardiac output. Pacemakers can be temporary or permanent, and there are many varieties, but they will not be covered in this book.

The nurse needs to be aware of where an external temporary pacemaker is available in his/her hospital in case one is needed in an emergency. Also, patients with a permanent pacemaker in place need to remember that their ECG will often look very different from a non-paced ECG trace because of the position of the pacing wire, which will affect the way that impulses pass across the myocardium.

Key learning points for *Chapter 3*

- In the acutely ill adult, heart rate, rhythm and strength should be monitored by feeling the patient's pulse and not via a measurement from an automatic reading device.

- Cardiac monitoring is helpful, but your assessment of 'how the patient is' comes before 'what is the rhythm?'

- Baroreceptors monitor stretch of the vascular system and respond to changes in blood pressure. They cause the system to constrict and dilate to maintain optimum blood pressure.

- Cardiac muscle cells have the intrinsic ability to contract without an external stimulus.

- The sino-atrial node is the main pacemaker of the heart and is stimulated by the vagus nerve.

- Shock has three stages. Early identification of shock can prevent further deterioration and possibly death.

- The patient may be in shock with a normal blood pressure (compensated shock).

- Central venous pressure readings are useful. The normal range is 3–8mmHg or 5–12cmH$_2$O.

Revision questions – cardiovascular

1. Name the cardiac rhythms shown in *Figures 3.13–3.15* and state what your actions would be with each.

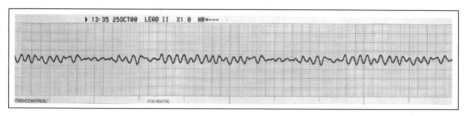

Figure 3.14: Revision ECG monitoring trace 1

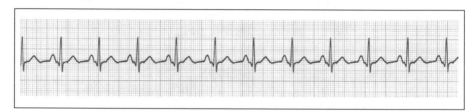

Figure 3.15: Revision ECG monitoring trace 2

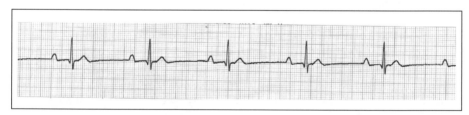

Figure 3.16: Revision ECG monitoring trace 3

2. Which nerve supplies the sino-atrial node in the heart?

3. Why are patients with atrial fibrillation given anticoagulation?

4. Where is the external pacemaker kept in your hospital?

Answers on page 197

References

Dellinger RP, Carlet JM, Masur H *et al* (2004) Surviving Sepsis Campaign guidelines for management of severe sepsis and septic shock. *Intensive Care Medicine* **30**(4): 536–535

Longmore M, Wilkinson I, Torok E (2001) *Oxford Handbook of Clinical Medicine*. 5th edn. Oxford University Press, Oxford

Swanton R (1998) *Cardiology*. 4th edn. Blackwell Science, Oxford

CHAPTER 4

Neurological care

P Pratt

This chapter will consider the neurological care of the acutely ill adult. For further information on this complex but important system, readers should consult the bibliography.

Assessment and observations

When assessing a patient for abnormal neurological function it is important to consider any recent neurological events and what has changed since the previous assessment (eg. is the patient still alert but with a new, reduced motor response, or is he/she now unconscious and responding only to pain).

Additional learning point

In the unconscious patient, remember Airway, Breathing and Circulation as the first point of assessment. Ensure that the patient is safe.

History

When assessing the course of events for the patient's deterioration, the nurse needs to be aware of the timescales involved in any neurological change. For example, was the patient sitting up chatting an hour ago but is now not rousable, or has he/she deteriorated slowly over the past few days? The following questions need to be posed:

- What is the patient normally like?
- Has the patient recently had a fall or sustained a head injury?

- Has a noisy patient become quiet?
- Has the patient complained of headaches or dizziness?
- Is there any history of neck stiffness or pain on head movement?
- Does the patient have a history of hypertension?
- Has a confused patient become drowsy?
- Is the patient orientated in time and place?

Basic observations

The nurse should record blood pressure, heart rate and rhythm, respiratory rate and pattern of breathing, and temperature; a random blood sugar measurement should also be checked if conscious level is affected. Other factors to consider are:

- Do the pupils respond equally and to light?
- Is the patient showing any new limb weakness or loss of sensation?

The nurse must assess the current state of consciousness and ensure that airway, breathing and circulation are maintained. A chart for recording the duration and frequency of seizures should be kept.

Glasgow coma scale and score

The Glasgow coma scale (GCS) score is the most common neurological assessment tool and reviews general global function. A score is generated from a possible total of 15. A GCS score of <8 is a very poor score, and indicates that the patient is at high risk, is unlikely to be able to maintain an adequate airway and may need further interventions. The GCS and scores are shown in *Table 4.1*.

Additional learning point
A significant deterioration in neurological function has occurred if the GCS score falls by 2 points or more.

Pupil reactions to light, vision and eye movements are dependent on normal functioning of the nerves that supply the eyes. Raised intracranial

Table 4.1: Glasgow coma scale and score*

Glasgow coma scale		Score
Eye opening response	Spontaneously	4
	To speech	3
	To pain	2
	None	1
Motor response	Obeys commands	6
	Localisation to painful stimulus	5
	Normal flexion to painful stimulus	4
	Spastic flexion to painful stimulus	3
	Extension to painful stimulus	2
	None	1
Verbal response	Orientated	5
	Confused	4
	Inappropriate words	3
	Incomprehensible sounds	2
	None	1
Total maximum score		**15**

*Record score for best response

pressure (ICP) or lesions involving the optic nerves may cause double vision, unequal or non-reactive pupils, loss of vision, abnormal gaze and abnormal movement of the eyes or eyelids. Drugs, eye diseases, and previous surgery also may affect eye observations.

Altered gaze and a change in pupil size and response must be reported urgently as a raised ICP needs to be managed quickly to prevent death.

Anatomy and physiology

It is important that the nurse caring for the acutely ill adult understands the basic anatomy and physiology of the nervous system. This vital system maintains homeostasis by the transmission of impulses along nerves to generate physiological responses. In this section we will consider the basic anatomical features of the nervous system.

The nervous system comprises the central nervous system (CNS) and the peripheral nervous system. The CNS consists of the brain and the spinal cord. The CNS connects with the peripheral nervous system, which consists of cranial nerves and spinal nerves, both of which have motor, sensory and autonomic components. We will also consider how impulses are passed along nerves and how synapses are formed. The most important issue for the nurse is to have an understanding of the physiology of the nervous system and its importance in the management of the acutely ill adult. The effects of the nervous system can be seen clinically in the way it impacts on other body systems.

Anatomy

The brain is one of the larger organs in the body. The main parts of the brain are the cerebrum, the cerebellum and the brainstem. The cerebrum is the largest part of the brain, and is made up of two halves termed hemispheres. Each hemisphere is divided into four lobes, known as the frontal, occipital, parietal and temporal lobes. The brainstem consists of the pons, the midbrain and the medulla. The brainstem continues down to form the spinal cord. The gross structures of the brain are shown in *Figure 4.1*.

The spinal cord extends down from the brainstem and has 30 pairs of nerves running from it. Nerve cells, termed neurones, make up the main body of nervous tissue. Each nerve cell consists of a cell body, an axon (carries impulses away from the cell) and several dendrites (receive impulses coming into the cell). In some but not all neurones, the outer layer of the axon is surrounded by a myelin sheath (allows impulses to travel

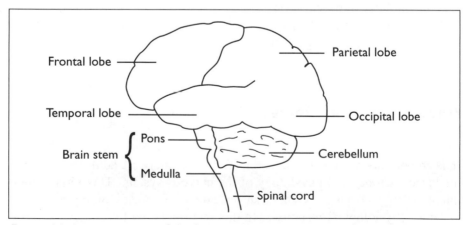

Figure 4.1: Basic anatomy of the brain

faster) (*Figure 4.2*). Impulses are transmitted from the CNS to the body via motor neurones, and from sensory receptors in the body to the CNS via sensory neurones.

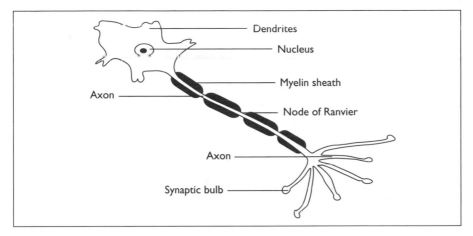

Figure 4.2: Basic anatomy of a neurone

Physiology

Covering the brain and extending to cover the spinal cord are three meninges (membranes): the dura mater, arachnoid mater and pia mater. The space between the arachnoid mater and pia mater contains the cerebrospinal fluid (CSF). CSF is important for the maintenance of homeostasis in the brain and spinal cord:

- It protects the brain and spinal cord from mechanical damage by acting as a cushion between the brain and skull.

- It maintains the optimal chemical environment for transmitting impulses from the brain and spinal cord to the other body systems.

- It acts as a medium for the exchange of waste and nutrients to and from the brain and spinal cord.

It is the CSF that is tested during a lumbar puncture; it should normally be clear fluid.

Transmission of a nerve impulse commences with the generation of an action potential in the nerve cell. When an action potential (impulse) is generated, it moves along the nerve axon to the synaptic bulb and transmitter substances are released from the synaptic bulb. These neurotransmitters cross the synapse

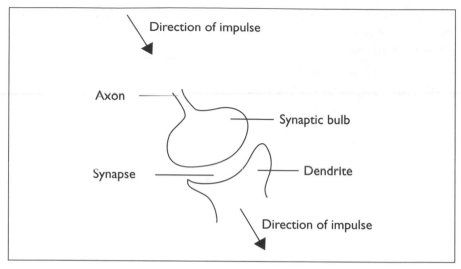

Figure 4.3: Diagram of a synapse

(*Figure 4.3*) and stimulate the dendrite of the next nerve, muscle or organ. There are thought to be at least 60 neurotransmitter substances, including the chemicals acetylcholine, norepinephrine (noradrenaline) and dopamine.

> Additional learning point
> Many drugs act at synaptic junctions, either blocking or accelerating the transmission of impulses to the next nerve, muscle or organ.

Many drugs that affect the brain act at these synapses. Also, many diseases affect the transmission of impulses at the synapse. Seizures are caused by the firing of excessive electrical impulses in the CNS, which are transmitted to other nerves and out to the skeletal muscles.

The sensory neurones of the peripheral nervous system carry impulses to the brain and spinal cord from the tissues and organs. These are interpreted by the brain and spinal cord, and messages are sent via the motor neurones of the peripheral nervous system to organs and tissues, which respond to these sensory findings.

The autonomic nervous system controls smooth muscle, cardiac muscle and some glands (exciting or inhibiting hormone excretion). The neurones of the autonomic system are divided into two groups: the parasympathetic system and the sympathetic system. These systems have no conscious control and act in opposition to maintain homeostasis.

> **Additional learning point**
> The autonomic nervous system maintains core functions and
> responds to acute illness, eg. by maintaining blood pressure and
> vital organ perfusion in the shocked patient through vasodilatation
> of vessels and an increase in heart rate.

Neurological diseases

Cerebrovascular accident (stroke)

Stroke may be defined as an event in which partial or complete loss of the
cerebral blood flow results in hypoxia and subsequent damage or death of
brain tissue. It has a rapid onset and lasts more than 24 hours. It occurs
secondary to either thromboembolism (ischaemic stroke) or cerebrovascular
haemorrhage (haemorrhagic stroke). Thus head injury as a cause of the
hypoxia is excluded.

Risk factors

* Hypertension
* Smoking
* Diabetes
* Obesity
* Hyperlipidaemia
* Heart disease.

Signs and symptoms

* Change in level of consciousness
* Aphasia (inability to speak)
* Dysphasia (difficulty in speech)
* Hemiplegia
* Dysphagia (difficulty in swallowing).

Key problems

The biggest concern in the context of the acutely ill adult is the initial management of consciousness and the patient's ability to maintain his/her own airway (see 'Care of the unconscious patient' later in this chapter).

Maintaining the patient's safety, giving anticonvulsants and ensuring that the airway is maintained, using adjuncts if necessary, are key challenges for the nurse.

Dysphagia may require the patient to be nil by mouth to prevent aspiration and associated complications.

Raised intracranial pressure

ICP is the pressure within the intracranial space. It is normally constant at around 0–15mmHg. If a person has a sneeze or cough, the ICP increases temporarily but returns to normal. If ICP rises too high, it attempts to displace the brain down into the spinal canal. This may eventually cause the brainstem to become hypoxic, and will lead to death if the pressure cannot be reduced. This movement of the brain tissue towards the spinal canal is called tentorial herniation or coning.

Risk factors

- Head injury
- Intracranial bleed
- Infection
- Hypoxia and hypercapnia
- Meninigitis

Signs and symptoms

- Change in level of consciousness
- Confusion
- Seizures
- Altered respiratory rate or rhythm
- Inability to regulate body temperature
- Diabetes insipidus (high urine output)

Key problems

It is very difficult to reduce a raised ICP, and the cause of the rise has to be identified. For example, a patient who has had a head injury and has an active bleed within the skull can be treated by neurosurgery (but not all bleeds can be treated in this way). However, if the raised ICP is secondary to infection and inflammation, treatments to reduce infection will be given to try to reduce the swelling and in turn the pressure. A raised ICP may give rise to a vast spectrum of problems, varying from a headache to unconsciousness and death.

Seizures

A seizure is a temporary but rapid contraction and relaxation of muscles that results in irregular and spasmodic movement of the limbs. A seizure is a symptom of an event occurring within the brain and may be related to a chronic condition or occur as a reaction to other illness. If a patient has a seizure, this does not necessarily mean that he/she is epileptic and will need long-term anticonvulsants.

> **Additional learning point**
> The occurrence of status epilepticus (multiple seizures without gaining consciousness, or a seizure lasting more than 20 minutes) in an acutely ill patient needs to be treated as an emergency and senior help called.
> The priority is to control the seizures.

Risk factors

- Family history
- Head injury
- Hypoxia
- Infection
- Hyperpyrexia
- Brain tumours
- Post stroke
- Drug treatments
- Metabolic disorders
- Eclampsia

Signs and symptoms

- The patient will have a rapid and sudden onset of spasmodic limb movements and be unresponsive to verbal or painful stimuli
- Urine or faecal incontinence
- Salivation, foaming at the mouth

Key problems

A seizure may be an indication of possible deterioration in the patient's condition, and progression of the severity of illness, especially in the context of the acutely ill adult with no history of seizures. Seizures also increase oxygen consumption and may worsen existing brain injury.

Meningitis

Meningitis is inflammation of the meninges of the brain and spinal cord. Meningitis must be treated urgently if suspected, as delay can result in death.

Risk factors

- Head injury
- Overcrowded areas, such as schools and colleges, increase the risk of transmission
- Immunocompromise
- Spinal anaesthesia
- Recent lumbar puncture

Signs and symptoms

- Headache
- Neck stiffness
- Photophobia
- Agitation
- Rash
- Vomiting
- Pyrexia

Not all of the above need to be present for meningitis to be suspected.

Key problems

- Symptoms may be of rapid onset
- Reduced consciousness
- Raised ICP
- Cardiovascular compromise
- Renal failure
- Sepsis
- Death

Treatments and interventions

Basics

- Airway and oxygen: Early assessment is vital in any patient with reduced consciousness or confusion. Oxygen should be prescribed and delivered by the most appropriate method, ie. one that the patient is most likely to be able to tolerate. This may be difficult in an agitated patient, and alternatives can be considered so that at least some oxygen is delivered.

- Positioning: It is important to position the patient to ensure optimum function and maintain the airway and breathing, particularly in an unconscious or semiconscious patient. The nurse should be able to put the patient into the recovery position when appropriate.

- GCS and core observations: Regular observations should be recorded and neurological observations checked. Any deterioration in the level of consciousness as indicated by a fall of 2 points or more on the GCS score must be reported to a senior member of staff and the patient fully assessed again.

Additional learning point
It is good practice, when handing over a patient to the next shift, to complete a set of neurological observations together to ensure that the same functions are measured and the baseline is agreed.

Care of the unconscious patient

If a patient is unconscious, regular observations must be recorded and parameters agreed with the clinical team as to what is acceptable. There are many causes of unconsciousness, and the cause in the individual patient should be established. A treatment plan must be in place to address both the cause of unconsciousness and management of the current state. Some patients become unconscious at the end of life and their treatment will often be less aggressive, but only acute care will be discussed in this section.

Care should include:

- Maintenance of a clear airway
- Possible use of airway adjuncts to maintain the airway
- Measures to reduce the risk of increasing ICP, such as:
  - avoid excessive coughing
  - position patient with head raised 45° if possible
- Regular observations, including blood pressure, heart rate, respiratory rate, oxygen saturation (SpO2) and temperature
- Blood glucose measurements
- Catheterisation and urine monitoring
- Pressure area care and positioning of limbs
- Meeting hydration and nutrition needs by the intravenous or enteral route as appropriate
- Implementation of the treatment plan in a timely way, e.g.
  - administer antibiotics on time
  - optimise oxygenation
  - manage any seizures or pain
  - ensure patient safety
- Oral and eye care
- Physiotherapy to prevent chest infection.

Drug treatments

Antibiotic therapy

The early administration of antibiotics is essential, particularly in the management of meningitis. Delays should not occur and doses must be administered on time in order to save lives and prevent disabilities.

The first-line antibiotic for the treatment of meningitis is ceftriaxone 4g stat, then ceftriaxone 2g once daily. Benzylpenicillin 1.2g can be given if no other antibiotics are available. Depending on the likely causative organism, other antibiotics may be used, but treatment should not be delayed until culture results are available. Check your local guidelines so that you know what is likely to be prescribed and how to administer it.

Anticonvulsant therapy

In this section, we will consider only drugs used for acute anticonvulsant therapy. Anticonvulsants are drugs that prevent and reduce seizures. Diazepam 10mg intravenously or 0.5mg/kg rectally may be given as a stat dose, and repeated as recommended in the British National Formulary (BNF). Respiratory compromise is possible and the patient must be closely monitored and observed.

If the patient continues to have seizures, the nurse must call for more senior help and reassess the patient. A patient with status epilepticus is likely to need a higher level of care than can be provided in a general ward environment.

Alternative methods of administering anticonvulsants must be arranged for patients who are nil by mouth, in order to maintain blood levels and reduce the risk of further seizure.

Advanced treatments and investigations

Lumbar puncture

A lumbar puncture is a procedure that allows a sample of CSF to be obtained, which can then be examined for infection. Lumbar puncture is not usually carried out if there is a suspicion of raised ICP, because of the risk of complications and death. It would also be contraindicated if there were any clotting abnormalities; a clotting screen should therefore be obtained if it is likely that a lumbar puncture may be considered.

After a lumbar puncture the patient may need to remain flat for a period of time (check local policy) and will need regular neurological observation using the GCS. Any deterioration in score or change in respiratory rate/rhythm, heart rate or blood pressure must be reported urgently as it may indicate a rise in ICP.

Key learning points for *Chapter 4*

- Remember the basics – airway, breathing and circulation must be assessed in the unconscious patient.

- The maximum Glasgow coma scale (GCS) score is 15 points. If a patient's GCS has fallen 2 points or more since the previous recording, further investigation is needed.

- Pupils should be equal and reacting to light.

- The brain has three meninges – the dura mater, arachnoid mater and pia mater. Cerebrospinal fluid occupies the space between the arachnoid and pia maters.

- Many drugs act at the synaptic junction between two neurones.

- Neurones can be sensory or motor.

- Seizures are not necessarily an indication of epilepsy and need further investigation, particularly in the acutely ill adult.

- As part of your assessment, check the blood glucose level in a patient whose conscious state has changed, even if the patient is not diabetic.

Revision questions – neurological

1. What is the maximum score that can be achieved using the GCS?

2. What is the priority in an unconscious patient?

3. Name the three meninges of the brain.

4. What is the most common antibiotic regimen used to treat bacterial meningitis?

Answers on page 197

Chapter 5

Renal care

P Pratt

Assessment and observations

History

A variety of signs and symptoms may suggest problems with renal function in the acutely ill adult. Some of the key concerns that should alert the nurse to the need for further investigations are:

- Reduced urine output
- Any use of diuretics
- Increased respiratory rate
- Cardiac arrhythmias
- Confusion or altered consciousness
- Pulmonary or peripheral oedema
- Nausea
- Diarrhoea and/or vomiting
- Electrolyte abnormalities, particularly urea, creatinine and potassium
- Recent episode of hypotension
- History of renal infections or stones

Assessment

Urine output

- What is the patient's urine output and is the patient catheterised?

If the patient is anuric, consider the possibility that the catheter may be blocked, or in the wrong position if it has just been inserted. It is important to act quickly to identify and correct any reduction in renal output. Terms that are commonly used to describe urine output are:

Oliguria	(urine output <300ml/24h)
Anuria	(urine output <100ml/24h)
Polyuria	(urine output >2000ml/24h)

However, the nurse should act within an hour or two of detecting a reduction in urine output (<0.5ml/kg/h), and not wait until the end of the 24-hour period.

- What does the urinalysis show?

All patients should have a urine sample tested with a dipstick on admission to obtain baseline values for renal function. Normal results are shown in *Table 5.1*.

Table 5.1 Normal dipstick urinalysis results

pH	4.5–8.0
Specific gravity	1.00–1.035
Protein	Negative
Glucose	Negative
Ketones	Negative
Bilirubin	Negative
Haemoglobin	Negative
White blood cells	Negative

The nurse should also note the odour and colour of the urine. Concentrated urine will often be dark and infective urine will usually have a foul smell. Urine is normally clear; if any odour, blood, pus or sediment is detected, a midstream sample should be sent for microbiology, culture and sensitivity. It is also possible to get a biochemical analysis of the sample. A 24-hour collection may be requested to give a full picture of renal function and how well electrolytes and waste products are being cleared by the kidneys.

> **Additional learning point**
> When using urine dipsticks, check the expiry date on the bottle and that
> they have been stored correctly.

If a patient has a 24-hour collection under way, it is only accurate if all the urine passed within the 24-hour period is collected. If one sample is missed, the collection must be restarted.

Observations

Urine output measurement and fluid balance

A fluid balance chart must be maintained for all acutely ill adults. Urine output is an indicator of renal function, and any change in volume above or below normal should raise concern in the nurse that it may be deteriorating. Similarly, a change in colour or smell of the urine should alert the nurse to the need for further investigation.

A fluid balance record must include both input and output of all fluids. It should be totalled at regular intervals and the balance recorded as either a positive or negative number. If urine output falls to <0.5ml/kg/h, it should be reassessed one hour later; if it is still <0.5/ml/kg/h, this finding should be reported to a senior member of staff. Hourly urine measurements and a strict fluid balance record should be commenced. See *Figure 1.2 (Chapter 1)* for an example of a fluid balance chart.

A fluid balance that is becoming increasingly positive should be reported if the patient starts to become wheezy, tachycardic or breathless. An accurate fluid balance should be presented at the medical ward round, along with all other care observations. A patient with a positive balance may not need any treatment, and intervention should only occur if problems are anticipated as a result of the increasing positive balance.

If the nurse asks for a medical review of an acutely ill patient, part of her regular observations should include an up-to-date fluid balance record. This is a vital part of assessment in the care of an acutely ill patient. The delivery of intravenous (IV) fluid in the acutely ill adult needs to be accurately maintained; it is therefore best to deliver all fluids via volumetric infusion devices where possible.

Fluid balance is important for the maintenance of homeostasis as body fluid makes up around 50–60% of total body weight. Body fluid is divided into two main compartments: intracellular and extracellular. Extracellular fluid is made up primarily of interstitial fluid and plasma.

Body fluid contains various solutes, nutrients, oxygen, proteins and electrolytes; these need to be regulated in order to maintain homeostasis. A change in the volume of body fluid can affect the balance of these solutes and have severe consequences for the acutely ill adult. In the well adult, this balance of fluid is maintained by a feedback loop (*Figure 5.1*).

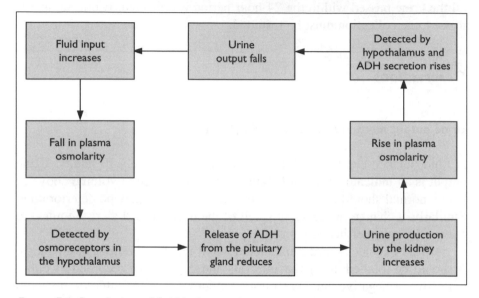

Figure 5.1: Regulation of fluid balance

Anatomy and physiology

Anatomy

The renal system, and predominantly the kidneys, has four main functions:

- Maintenance of fluid balance
- Regulation of acid-base homeostasis and other electrolytes
- Removal of waste products of metabolism
- Production of erythropoietin and vitamin D.

Most people have two kidneys, two ureters, one bladder and one urethra.

Some patients may have only one kidney or one functioning kidney and can manage very well in normal health; however, if they become unwell they will be particularly susceptible to renal problems. Blood flow to the kidney is via the renal artery into the body of the kidney; the renal artery then divides into smaller arterioles, each of which divides to give a network of capillaries (the glomerulus) through which plasma is delivered to the kidney for filtering. Twenty-five per cent of cardiac output is delivered to the kidneys, ie. >1000ml/min. A complex mechanism of dilatation and relaxation of the blood vessels regulates blood flow and pressure in the kidneys. The main functional unit of the kidney is the nephron (*Figure 5.2*).

Within the glomerulus of the nephron, blood is filtered across membranes: the hydrostatic pressure forces water and small molecules (<70000 daltons) through the endothelial fenestrations into the capsular space. Large molecules such as albumin and some colloids cannot normally pass into the capsular space and remain in the circulatory system. The resulting fluid in the capsular space is called the glomerular filtrate.

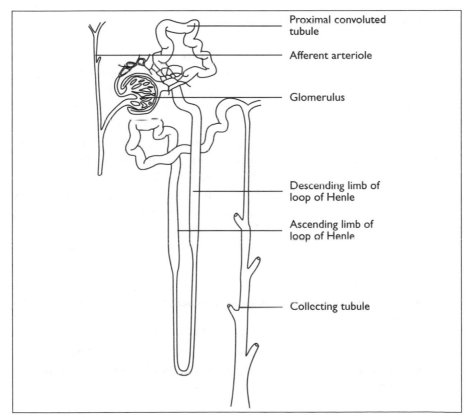

Figure 5.2: Basic anatomy of a nephron

Physiology

The body of the kidney contains many nephrons, which perform filtration, re-absorption and secretion. These functions maintain homeostasis of the blood. Waste products are excreted in the urine and other substances are reabsorbed.

To ensure that filtration occurs, blood pressure within the kidney needs to be maintained. Fluid is pushed into the capsular space under pressure. Selective reabsorption of water and electrolytes then takes place in the remainder of the nephron (tubules and collecting duct). Maintenance of adequate blood pressure is vital for kidney function.

Raised intra-abdominal pressure may reduce renal blood flow and compromise renal function. Obstruction of the ureters or bladder may also compromise renal function by raising the pressure in the urinary system.

Factors affecting glomerular filtration rate

Around 18% of blood volume enters the renal capsule each day, and approximately 180 litres of glomerular filtrate is produced; however, most of the filtrate is reabsorbed, with only 1–2% of it excreted as urine. The kidney's ability to filter the blood entering the renal capsule by forcing substances through the endothelial fenestration is dependent on blood pressure. Glomerular filtration rate (GFR) in a normal adult is approximately 125ml/min and a critical fall in systemic blood pressure, regardless of cause, will decrease the blood flow through the kidney. Although some compensation can be achieved by autoregulatory vasoconstriction, renal blood pressure will eventually fall, and hence GFR will decrease.

In the acutely ill patient, a fall in blood pressure can directly affect renal function. However, patients are able to compensate by the intrinsic responses of the negative feedback system that optimise GFR by autoregulation. If a fall in blood pressure is detected within the renal circulation, renin is released into the blood. This converts a chemical called angiotensinogen to angiotensin-I. Angiotensin-I is then converted to angiotensin-II, which has a number of effects (*Table 5.2*). Once normal blood pressure is achieved, the negative feedback process inhibits the release of renin and its effects cease.

Table 5.2: Effects of angiotensin-II release

Vasoconstriction of arterioles	Increases systemic vascular resistance, which in turn raises mean arterial blood pressure
Stimulation of aldosterone secretion from the adrenal cortex	Increases the retention of sodium ions (Na+) and chloride ions (Cl-), and hence water, by the kidneys
Stimulation of thirst centre	Makes the patient feel thirsty and want to increase oral fluid intake
Stimulation of antidiuretic hormone (ADH) secretion from the posterior pituitary gland	Increases water retention

> Additional learning point
> Angiotensin-converting enzyme (ACE) inhibitors act on the renin-angiotensin system and may be used to treat hypertension.

Disease of the capillary walls sometimes allows proteins to enter the glomerular filtrate; this causes a rise in osmotic pressure within the renal capsule, and as a result extra water is drawn in. Protein can also be found in the urine when infection is present. Therefore, when the nurse checks a urinalysis and finds that protein has been detected in the urine of an acutely ill patient, this should alert him/her to the need for further investigation.

Tubular reabsorption

Around 98% of glomerular filtrate is reabsorbed. However, this tubular reabsorption has to be selective if the functions of the kidney are to be achieved. Most of the filtered substances are reabsorbed (Table 5.3) and only 1% of the filtrate is excreted as urine.

Table 5.3: Substances reabsorbed from the nephron

Glucose	Potassium	Phosphate
Amino acids	Calcium	Proteins
Urea	Chloride	Peptides
Sodium	Bicarbonate	Water

Acid-base balance and the kidney

The kidneys' ability to excrete hydrogen ions and retain bicarbonate ions is crucial to the maintenance of acid-base homeostasis. This compensation system works in conjunction with the respiratory system to control acid-base balance. If the respiratory system is not able to compensate, as in a patient with respiratory failure, for example, carbon dioxide may be retained and a respiratory acidosis will develop. The first response will be an increase in respiratory rate, but if this does not correct pH then the renal system will try to compensate. The excretion or retention of hydrogen ions allows the blood pH to be maintained within the range 7.35–7.45. The renal system compensates for a reduced pH (acidosis) by increasing the excretion of hydrogen ions. These attach to bicarbonate ions and are excreted in the form of carbonic acid, making the urine more acid. There is also reabsorption and increased production of bicarbonate ions, which neutralise acid and maintain the pH within normal limits. Bicarbonate is therefore an acid buffer. The respiratory system compensates for changes in pH by altering the pattern of breathing. This is called respiratory compensation.

Renal diseases

Renal failure

Acutely ill adults are at risk of developing renal failure and it is important for the nurse caring for this group of patients to be aware of the signs and symptoms of acute renal failure. Early intervention can reverse disease progression and minimise the risk of long-term renal failure.

Renal failure is a reduction in glomerular filtration, leading to an inability to excrete waste products and maintain fluid and acid-base balance. It is life-threatening and early management is vital. Diagnosis is confirmed by testing a blood sample and further investigation, but the nurse can note signs and symptoms.

The main abnormalities used to confirm acute renal failure are:

- Raised urea and creatinine in the blood
- Hyperkalaemia
- Metabolic acidosis
- Oliguria.

All of these abnormalities occur as the kidney becomes unable to filter waste products. Renal failure may be acute or chronic, and can be caused by several different factors. These may be divided into three groups:

- Pre-renal causes: A fall in blood pressure and a reduction in renal perfusion secondary to a reduction in cardiac output or hypovolaemia can lead to renal failure. Causes of the fall in cardiac output need to be examined, and were discussed in the cardiovascular section (*Chapter 3*). Irreversible renal failure will occur if ongoing hypotension is not corrected quickly.

- Renal causes: Damage to the epithelial lining of the renal tubules can be caused by drugs, heavy metal poisoning, infections or other systemic diseases, and is often chronic. Pre-renal failure can lead to established renal failure.

- Post-renal causes: These are related to an obstruction, such as tumour or renal stones, that initially block the drainage of urine. The blockage leads to a rise in pressure in the kidney tubules and so prevents filtration occurring, causing irreversible damage. Renal failure may take longer to become established with an obstructive cause, and may be unilateral and go undetected as the healthy kidney compensates. If post-renal obstruction is relieved in time, renal function may recover.

Risk factors

- Low blood pressure
- Hypovolaemia
- Shock
- Sepsis (causes both renal and pre-renal failure)
- Poor renal perfusion

- Reduction in cardiac output
- Urological disease

Signs and symptoms

- Oliguria
- Anuria
- Elevated or rising urea and creatinine
- Hyperkalemia
- Metabolic acidosis
- Increased respiratory rate

Key problems

Untreated renal failure may lead to death. Short-term management includes control of electrolyte abnormality, especially hyperkalaemia, and control of fluid balance. Haemofiltration or dialysis may be needed to control electrolytes and fluid balance and remove waste substances.

The acutely ill patient is at high risk of renal dysfunction, and the nurse should ensure that urine output is monitored on any patient who is at risk of becoming acutely unwell.

Treatments and interventions

Basics

- Strict record of fluid balance
- Monitoring of urine output
- Catheterisation
- Monitoring of urea, creatinine and serum potassium levels
- Review of medication that may effect renal function

Additional learning point
A reduction in urine output to <0.5ml/kg/h for more than 2 hours should be reported and investigated further, and steps should be taken to treat the cause.

When a patient has a reduced renal function, any drugs that are nephrotoxic (harmful to the kidney) need to be stopped. Dose reduction may be necessary for certain drugs that are excreted via the kidney. The ward pharmacist can advise you on this. Examples of common nephrotoxic drugs include:

- Gentamicin
- Non-steroidal anti-inflammatory drugs
- ACE inhibitors.

Fluid and electrolyte monitoring

It is important to monitor all electrolytes in the acutely ill patient, but we will consider specifically hyperkalaemia as potassium is the first electrolyte to be influenced by renal dysfunction, and small changes from normal levels may have profound effects on all organ systems.

Hyperkalaemia

Hyperkalaemia (elevated potassium in the blood) alters the membrane potential of nerves and muscle, and therefore affects cardiac and neuromuscular function. Cardiac monitoring should be commenced in a patient with hyperkalaemia as arrhythmias are common (particularly atrial fibrillation and ectopic beats). If the blood potassium level is >6.5mmol/litre, a widened QRS segment and peaked T-waves may be seen on ECG and the patient is at risk of cardiac arrest.

If the patient has other electrolyte disturbances, such as hypocalcaemia, hypomagnesaemia, acidaemia or hyponatraemia (low blood sodium level), the effects of hyperkalaemia will be more severe.

Treatments for hyperkalaemia: Potassium excretion can be increased by loop diuretics such as furosemide. Potassium intake should be reduced; potassium-free IV fluids, eg. dextrose or saline, should be given. Dextrose and insulin administration will facilitate the uptake of potassium into the cells, decreasing the serum potassium concentration. Rectal or oral potassium-absorbing resin preparations may be given to bind potassium from the gastrointestinal system. IV administration of calcium chloride will temporarily protect the heart from the effects of severe hyperkalaemia. Referral for haemofiltration or dialysis may be needed.

Drugs

Diuretics such as furosemide are commonly used on acute wards to increase urine output. They can be given orally, by IV bolus or by continuous IV infusion. Diuretics may increase urine output even if the patient is hypovolaemic and should not be given without assessing the patient's hydration status. It is crucial to carry out a full assessment of the patient's fluid balance status in order to exclude causes of low cardiac output and hence poor renal perfusion.

Additional learning point
In postoperative surgical patients, a urine output of <0.5ml/kg/h is almost always due to hypovolaemia, therefore hypovolaemia should be excluded before administering a diuretic.

Advanced interventions and treatments

Intravenous access

In patients with severe renal dysfunction who are acutely ill it is common to insert a central venous catheter in order to manage and optimise fluid balance. The nurse should consult the cardiovascular section (Chapter 3) for details on central lines.

Dialysis

Renal replacement therapy can be given in the form of dialysis. This is generally carried out in areas providing higher levels of care, such as high dependency units or intensive care units, and will not be discussed in this book.

Indications for acute dialysis are:

- Hyperkalaemia
- Fluid overload
- Severe metabolic acidosis.

Key learning points for *Chapter 5*

- Minimum acceptable urine output is 0.5ml/kg/h

- Fluid balance records must include input and output of all fluids.

- A fall in blood pressure will directly affect renal blood pressure and in turn affect urine output.

- The kidneys maintain blood pH by excreting and retaining hydrogen and bicarbonate ions.

- The causes of renal failure are divided into three categories: pre-renal, renal and post-renal. The acutely ill patient is at most risk from pre-renal causes.

- Some medications affect the kidney and should be discontinued or administered in a reduced dose in a patient with impaired renal function. Check the drugs that your patient has been prescribed with your ward pharmacist if you are unsure.

- Furosemide is rarely used to treat oliguria in the surgical patient.

Revision questions – renal case study

Fred Jones is a 42-year-old man who underwent a hemicolectomy 2 days ago. He has a history of hypertension and his regular medication includes lisinopril 5mg. His observations that you recorded this morning are:

Heart rate	110 beats/min
Blood pressure	105/65mmHg
Respiratory rate	18 breaths/min
Temperature	37°C
Urine output	135ml since the bag was last emptied

He is alert and tells you he feels thirsty. He has been on 4-hourly observations and his fluid chart was discontinued at 12pm last night after his catheter was emptied.

1. What nursing interventions will you carry out?
2. When will you next complete a set of observations?
3. What are your initial concerns?
4. What other information will you want to collect?

Answers on page 198

CHAPTER 6

Gastrointestinal care

P Pratt

Assessment and observations

History

A gastrointestinal history includes questioning about various aspects of gastrointestinal function from the mouth to the anus. The history usually follows the direction indicated by a particular complaint or observed circumstance. Chewing and swallowing at the mouth, where food is mixed with salivary digestive juices and broken down into a soft thick liquid for swallowing, are the start of the digestive process.

The following symptoms are important pointers to problems with gastrointestinal function and require further investigation:

* Difficulty in swallowing
* Dry mouth
* Oral odour
* Frequent episodes of choking and coughing during or after eating.

Chest pain and heartburn from indigestion or hiatus hernia with gastro-oesophageal reflux can mimic angina pectoris and may radiate to the neck, the back or the left arm and hand. Persistent hiccoughs may be caused by oesophageal reflux, or by irritation of the diaphragm due to a subphrenic abscess.

Pain or a burning sensation in the stomach area may indicate gastritis or peptic ulcer. Pain in the hypochondrium may also come from the liver capsule or the gallbladder. Pain may be constant or episodic and may be associated with nausea and vomiting. Its onset, duration, location, precipitating or relieving factors, and intensity should be noted.

Vomiting, with details of frequency, content, appearance and volume, should be noted. Abdominal swelling or masses, or generalised distension, should be recorded. Appetite and bowel habits should be documented; frequency, appearance and odour of stools, constipation or straining, pain, and the passage of flatus are also pertinent aspects of the gastrointestinal history. Blood per rectum may be fresh or the tarry, foul-smelling melaena (stools) containing digested blood from the upper gastrointestinal tract.

A gastrointestinal history must therefore include a record of the onset, frequency and duration of the following symptoms and signs, and other relevant information:

- Appetite, food and fluid intake, past and more recent
- Indigestion
- Choking or difficulty in swallowing
- Nausea and vomiting
- Pain or cramps
- Abdominal distension, masses or swellings
- Previous or recent surgery
- Bowel habits, constipation or diarrhoea
- Flatulence.

Assessment

Assessment begins with gaining a clear history from the patient or family. What the nurse observes, the current condition of the patient and the effect that his/her gastrointestinal symptoms are having on other systems are important in the context of the acutely ill adult. Listen, look and palpate. General aspects to consider during your assessment should include global signs such as pallor, which may indicate anaemia from bleeding, or jaundice from liver disease or biliary obstruction. Other specific assessments should include:

- Is the patient eating and drinking, or is enteral or parenteral feeding being administered?

- Is the patient nauseous or vomiting? What is the likely cause and can it be treated? What is the volume, content and frequency of vomiting?

- Is the patient's bowel function regular? What is the stool colour, volume and frequency of defecation?

- Is the patient passing large amounts of loose stool? If so, this may lead to fluid balance deficits, and possibly electrolyte imbalance if the draining fluid is high in potassium.

- Does the patient have any abdominal distension? If so, is this affecting other body systems? For example, the respiratory system and breathing can be affected: a distended abdomen can cause splinting of the diaphragm and lead to basal atelectasis or collapse, or in severe cases respiratory failure. This is of particular concern in the patient whose respiratory function is already compromised, or who has chronic respiratory disease. If abdominal distension becomes severe, the increased intra-abdominal pressure may lead to a reduction in kidney perfusion and eventually renal failure. Distension may be measured using a tape measure to record the circumference of the abdomen, or using transduced bladder pressure to determine intra-abdominal pressure.

- The volume of drainage fluid, either post-surgery or from the drainage of ascites, is important: a large volume may indicate hypovolaemia, with implications for the circulatory and renal systems, and a low volume may indicate that the drain is no longer necessary and should be removed.

- Pain needs to be assessed as it may impact on breathing if a patient is unable to cough and remove lung secretions. The patient will then be at risk of developing pneumonia. Pain assessment is discussed in detail in *Chapter 8*.

Additional learning point
More things are missed in the acutely ill adult by not looking rather than by not knowing.

Observations

- The abdomen impacts on other organ systems – the respiratory system and breathing, the circulatory system, the renal system etc – and observations pertaining to one system may impact on or reflect the function or status of other systems. The nurse should therefore complete a full set of observations, including respiratory rate, blood pressure, heart rate, urine output, conscious level and saturation of oxygen, when assessing the acutely ill patient.

- Detailed assessment of respiratory function should be carried out, as chest infections and pneumonia are common complications in patients with abdominal pain. Respiratory rate, depth of breathing and ability to cough should all be assessed.

- Fluid balance records should be reviewed and the volumes of fluid intake and output, and the frequencies of intake and output from feeding and/or drainage, recorded.

- Abdominal distension, in terms of either abdominal circumference or intra-abdominal pressure, may be measured and recorded.

- The process of swallowing may be affected by degenerative disease or stroke, and lead to choking and aspiration. Patients with a tracheostomy or who have recently been extubated and transferred from intensive care may have inadequate swallowing and a swallowing assessment may be necessary. The need for a swallowing assessment will be dependent on local policy, and the individual circumstances of the patient should be assessed to ensure the safety of the airway. If in doubt, keep the patient nil by mouth until an assessment has been carried out.

Anatomy and physiology

Anatomy

The gastrointestinal system extends from the mouth down via the oesophagus to the stomach, into the small bowel, which consists of the duodenum, the jejunum and the ileum. It continues along into the large bowel, consisting of the caecum, the ascending, transverse, descending and sigmoid colon, and the rectum, and ends at the anus. Other organs, namely the liver, gallbladder and pancreas, connect to the duodenum via the common bile duct (*Figure 6.1*). The spleen has no gastrointestinal function, but is mentioned here because it occurs within the abdomen and because it and its blood supply lie in close proximity to other gastrointestinal organs. The kidneys and adrenal glands are retroperitoneal organs, which may be palpable or tender, causing abdominal symptoms and signs.

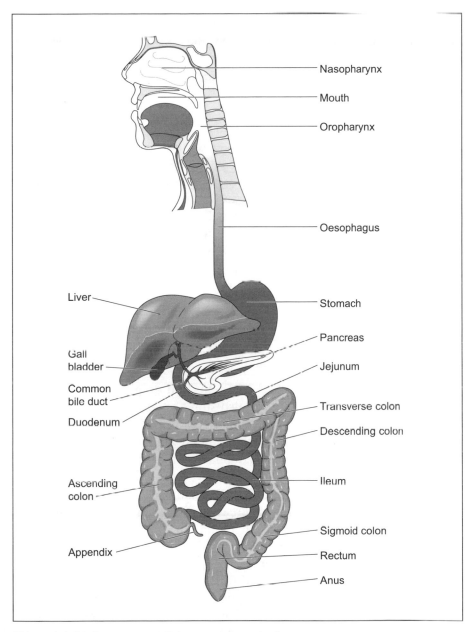

Figure 6.1 Basic anatomy of the gastrointestinal tract

Physiology

The oral cavity opens at the lips of the mouth and contains the teeth and the tongue. Food is chewed in the oral cavity (this process is termed mastication) to break it down into small particles, and mixed with salivary enzymes before being swallowed. The mouth or oropharynx communicates with the nasopharynx, which is isolated during swallowing by the soft palate. The pharyngeal constrictor muscles provide a coordinated contraction, forcing food or fluid downwards into the oesophagus, while simultaneously isolating the airways and vocal cords during swallowing.

The oesophagus then forces the food bolus downwards into the stomach. The pH in the stomach is acidic and should normally be <5.5; this can be altered by drug administration and is discussed further in the nutrition section (*Chapter 7*). In the stomach, gastric digestive juices are mixed with the food to form chyme. The chyme is forced, in small amounts, by peristaltic movements, through the pyloric valve into the duodenum, where further digestive juices from the liver, gallbladder and pancreas are added from the common bile duct. Nutrients, fluids and medications are absorbed from the gastrointestinal mucosa. Different nutrients and vitamins may be absorbed from different locations in the gastrointestinal tract. Most absorption takes place in the jejunum and ileum as the gastrointestinal content passes along, by peristalsis, until it reaches the rectum where it awaits defecation through the anus. The content of the small bowel is usually sterile, but the large bowel and rectum contain large numbers of bacteria. The small bowel joins the large bowel at the ileocaecal junction, where the appendix is also located.

The liver modifies substances (nutrients and drugs or poisons) and is the main organ of detoxification. It also stores and synthesizes substances for the body. The liver has a dual blood supply – it receives blood from the systemic circulation and also from the gut via the portal veins, which carry nutrients (and drugs) to be metabolised before entry into the systemic circulation via the hepatic veins. The liver excretes bile, and certain substances excreted in the bile may be reabsorbed by the gut during the enterohepatic circulation. The pancreas also has an endocrine function and produces insulin, which controls blood glucose concentration and the absorption of glucose by the tissues.

Some drugs are absorbed in the stomach, others are absorbed in the small bowel, and some may be absorbed directly from the mucosa in the mouth (sublingual administration) or the rectum (as with rectal suppository). The oral doses of many drugs are larger than the intravenous doses because of the first-pass effect, which results in a proportion of the drug absorbed from the stomach or intestine being inactivated by the liver before entering the systemic circulation; for example, the oral dose for atenolol is 25–100mg, whereas the intravenous dose is not more than 5mg.

Gastrointestinal diseases

The treatment for many gastrointestinal conditions in the acutely ill patient may need to be surgery. In an already ill person, this a serious demand to make of his/her physiological reserves and is not to be undertaken lightly, especially if the diagnosis is unsure or may respond to conservative management. There is much overlap in the general management of surgical patients: the core components of care focus on adequate hydration, general care and monitoring the progress of the interventions instigated. Regular monitoring of the condition of the patient and responding to signs and symptoms from all organ systems is a challenge for the nurse.

Peptic ulcer disease

Gastric or duodenal ulcer may be defined as a defect in the mucosa of the stomach or duodenum.

Symptoms

* Pain or burning in the epigastrium.

Risks

* Bleeding
* Perforation

Key problems

The risk of erosion of a blood vessel leading to a major bleed should not be underestimated. It is useful to remember that acutely ill adults, and elderly people in particular, may develop 'stress ulcers'; proton pump inhibitors or histamine-H$_2$ receptor antagonists may often be given as preventive therapy.

Acute abdomen

The acute abdomen is characterised by:

- Sudden or recent onset of pain; the pain is usually constant
- Peritonitis resulting from infection and irritation of the peritoneum
- Rebound tenderness
- Abdominal muscle guarding
- Severe pain; the patient will lie as still as possible
- Loss of appetite and often vomiting
- Reduced or absent bowel sounds
- The abdomen may be distended
- Patient may be anaemic or in shock
- Patient may exhibit signs of sepsis, ie. pyrexia, tachycardia or hypotension.

Acute abdomen may be caused by infection, haemorrhage into the peritoneal space, or perforation. It may originate in the gynaecological organs, as in ruptured ectopic pregnancy or infection of the female organs. Patients with an acute abdomen will require surgery for removal of the source of the infection, which may cause sepsis and death if left. Resection of diseased or damaged bowel may be needed. Other conditions that may present as an acute abdomen will now be considered.

Acute bowel obstruction

Bowel obstruction consists of blockage of the bowel. It can be caused by a mechanical factor within the bowel lumen, the bowel wall or outside the bowel.

Risk factors

- Adhesions, possibly from previous surgery
- Tumour of the bowel

- Sigmoid volvulus
- A mass outside the bowel or infiltrating the bowel

Symptoms and signs

- Possible history of previous surgery
- Distension
- Constipation
- Absent flatus
- Loss of appetite
- Nausea and vomiting
- Colicky-type pain
- Tender abdomen
- Usually apyrexial without signs of sepsis

Key problems

- Vomiting
- Fluid balance
- Abdominal distension

Pancreatitis

Pancreatitis is defined as inflammation of the pancreas. It has three main causes (listed below). Severity of pancreatitis is diagnosed using Ranson's criteria (*Table 6.1*): a patient with three or more of these criteria is deemed to have severe pancreatitis. The criteria cannot be applied fully until 48 hours after admission and are a poor predictor later in the disease. Pancreatitis carries at least 10% mortality, and the more points on the Ranson criteria a patient has, the worse the prognosis.

Risk factors

- Viral infection
- Obstruction of the common bile duct, usually by gallstone but can be tumour
- Alcohol abuse

Table 6.1: Ranson's criteria* for predicting mortality in pancreatitis

On admission	Age >55 years
	White cell count >16 x 10^9/litre
	Lactate dehydrogenase (LDH) >350iu/litre
	Aspartate transaminase (AST) >60iu/litre
	Blood glucose >11mmol/litre
Within 48 hours of admission	Haematocrit fall >10%
	Urea rise >10mmol/litre
	Serum calcium <2mmol/litre
	Base excess >-4
	PaO$_2$ <8kPa
	Estimated fluid sequestration >6 litres

Source: London and Hemingway (2005)

Signs and symptoms

- Abdominal distension
- Pain and upper abdominal tenderness
- Absent bowel sounds
- Loss of appetite, vomiting
- Raised serum amylase levels
- Apyrexial usually, unless infected cyst or other infection is present
- May exhibit signs of systemic inflammatory response syndrome (SIRS)

Key problems

- The pancreas produces digestive enzymes; if these leak out of the pancreatic ducts they may damage the pancreatic tissue itself and cause generalised tissue necrosis.

- The formation of pseudocysts; these may become infected and cause sepsis, or if large may give rise to mechanical problems such as abdominal distension.

- Patients who are misdiagnosed and undergo surgery (laparotomy) do worse than those who do not have surgery.

■ Associated problems can be complex, and include problems with malnutrition and immune compromise.

■ Renal function may be compromised as a result of infection, raised intra-abdominal pressure and fluid balance inadequacies.

■ A distended abdomen and pain will impact on breathing.

■ Patients with pancreatitis often have hypovolaemia due to ascites and sequestration of a large fluid volume.

■ In severe cases the patient will suffer major haemorrhage, develop shock and may die.

United Kingdom guidelines for the management of acute pancreatitis (1998) detail the best practice management for this high-risk group of patients.

Diverticular disease

Diverticular disease is the formation of small sacs of herniation of the large bowel mucosa through a weakening in the bowel wall. It may lead to infective episodes of acute diverticulitis.

Risk factors

• Poor fibre intake
• Increasing age (greater in those aged >80 years)

Signs and symptoms

• Abdominal pain and tenderness
• Tachycardia
• Pyrexia
• Acute abdomen
• Diverticular mass

Key problems

- Bowel perforation (see below)
- Obstruction of the bowel
- Bleeding

Surgery may be necessary. As this is often performed in older patients with co-morbidities, there is a significant risk of death. This group of patients requires close observation and management and present a challenge for the ward nurse.

Bowel perforation

Bowel perforation may be described as an interruption of the integrity of the full thickness of the bowel wall with escape of intestinal content and air into the peritoneal cavity, usually causing an acute abdomen.

Risk factors

- Bowel obstruction
- Foreign body within the bowel, such as a bone
- Ulceration
- Diverticulitis
- Tumour

Signs and symptoms

- Acute abdomen
- Sepsis, pyrexia
- Vomiting
- Distended abdomen

Key problems

Patients with bowel perforation often develop peritonitis and may end up with severe infection and sepsis.

Intra-abdominal haemorrhage

Intra-abdominal haemorrhage is defined as bleeding into the abdominal cavity.

Risk factors

- Post surgery
- Abdominal aortic aneurysm
- Ectopic pregnancy
- Trauma

Signs and symptoms

- Tachycardia
- Hypotension
- Peritonitis/acute abdomen
- Fall in urine output
- Retroperitoneal haematoma

Key problems

In this condition, large volumes of blood may be lost with no visible outward sign; the nurse must therefore be aware of compensatory mechanisms (eg. tachycardia) that signify early shock. Worsening pain, a fall in urine output and a raised respiratory rate should all ring alarm bells. A fall in blood pressure is a late sign which signifies that normal compensatory mechanisms are failing and urgent intervention is needed.

Treatments and interventions

Basics

- Infection control: Strict attention to gloving, hand-washing and cleanliness is essential because gastrointestinal secretions often have high bacterial counts and must not be allowed to contaminate clean areas.

■ Observations: Patients who have undergone a major surgical procedure will need special care and vigilance during the postoperative phase because of the possibility of early or late complications. If these occur, timely intervention will reduce unnecessary suffering.

■ Pain relief: A balance must be found between the provision of adequate analgesia and the potential side-effects of analgesic drugs and their methods of administration. For example, opiates may cause unwanted respiratory depression in those who are already at risk of lung complications due to surgery. Local anaesthetics given by the epidural route may increase the risk of hypotension. These issues are addressed more fully in the section on pain management (*Chapter 8*).

Nasogastric tube

Nasogastric tubes present a number of problems and potential dangers:

• They can be uncomfortable for the patient.
• They may be pulled out accidentally and have to be re-inserted.
• The nurse must ensure that the correct siting of the tube has been confirmed, ie. it is positioned in the stomach and not curled in the throat or in the bronchial tree. The administration of medications, fluid or feed through a tube that is not in the stomach or duodenum can have disastrous effects, eg. chemical pneumonitis.
• The tube may become blocked.

Nil by mouth

Patients may need to be kept nil by mouth for several reasons:

• As part of the management of their condition
• Because they are awaiting surgery
• Because oral intake may be undesirable as a result of recent surgery.

Nil-by-mouth orders need to be clear, as oral intake may lead to cancelled operations or vomiting if incorrectly allowed. Conversely, it may be unfair to withhold oral intake when this is unnecessary.

Drug treatments

Anti-emetics

Anti-emetics are commonly used in general wards to relieve the side-effects of other drugs or to treat the symptoms of illness. Metoclopramide, cyclizine, prochlorperazine and ondansetron are frequently prescribed to relieve nausea and vomiting, and can be given by a variety of routes.

Antacids

Antacids are used in the treatment and prevention of peptic ulcer disease. Examples include ranitidine and proton pump inhibitors. Gaviscon may be given for symptomatic relief.

Key learning points for *Chapter 6*

- Remember to ascertain whether the patient has any problems with eating or appetite, and whether these problems are new or longstanding.

- Does the patient look pale or jaundiced? This may need further investigation.

- Remember to get a bowel habit history and collect a stool specimen if any unusual odour, mucus or diarrhoea is present.

- A distended or painful abdomen will affect the ability of other body systems to function effectively. Patients with abdominal pain are very susceptible to chest infections and respiratory failure.

- Acutely ill patients are at risk of developing stress ulcers. The nurse should consider this possibility if new complaints of gastric pain are reported.

- Patients with pancreatitis need close observation and careful monitoring of other body systems, including fluid balance. They are at risk of significant deterioration and the nurse should report any signs of shock or infection.

Revision questions – gastroenterology

1. Why do patients with abdominal pain have an increased risk of developing respiratory failure?

2. What is the pH in the stomach?

3. List the three main causes of pancreatitis.

4. List two ways to measure abdominal distension.

Answers on page 198

References

London N, Hemingway D (2005) *University Hospitals of Leicester NHS Surgical Handbook*. Surgical Directorate

United Kingdom guidelines for the management of acute pancreatitis. British Society of Gastroenterology (1998) *Gut* **42**(Suppl 2): S1–13

CHAPTER 7

Nutrition

J Kennedy

Nutrition is defined as the food one eats and the way in which the body uses it for proper body functioning, survival, growth, repair of worn-out tissues and maintenance of health. Conversely, malnutrition may describe any disorder concerning nutrition. It may result from an unbalanced, insufficient or excessive diet or the impaired absorption, assimilation or use of foods. Consequently, visual observation of an individual to determine nutritional status is not enough.

Undernutrition is common in hospitals (McWhirter and Pennington, 1994). In the hospital setting, the patient's illness and associated morbidity, in addition to environmental factors, put him/her at higher risk of developing undernutrition, or of being undernourished and it going unnoticed and thus untreated, compared with his/her peers in the community. Up to 40% of patients in intensive care units receive no nutritional support (Heyland *et al*, 2003) and so return to the ward environment already in a weakened state.

Assessment of nutritional status

The aims of nutritional assessment are to:

- Assess the risk of morbidity and mortality resulting from protein-energy malnutrition
- Identify the causes and consequences of undernutrition and disease in the individual
- Ascertain whether the patient will benefit clinically from nutritional support.

Nutritional screening should address issues such as the patient's recent, unintentional weight loss, reduced appetite, eating or digestive difficulties, energy expenditure, fatigue and the presence of other factors such as infection, ongoing disease process, radiotherapy, pain and recent surgery.

Nutritional status has traditionally been defined in terms of weight, variations in weight, body mass index, plasma protein concentration, immune competence and observation of patient's dietary intake, coupled with assessment of variation from normal intake as a result of illness and assessment of functional change. Functional impairment and changes in body composition are of equal importance and interlinked.

Weight is a good longitudinal measure of nutritional status, with severe malnutrition defined as actual body weight ≤70% of ideal weight for height. Unplanned weight loss of >10% over a 3-month period is often a good indicator of poor outcome. However, it would be incorrect to take body weight in isolation and to base aggressive nutritional intervention on it. It is important to determine the patient's 'dry weight' and the amount of oedema present, as oedema (and obesity) may mask the loss of lean body mass and potential malnutrition. Body weight can fluctuate, rise or fall with nutritional and fluid intake or lack of it, with renal, liver, thyroid or cardiac impairment, and with the effects of medication. Comparison of the patient's weight with charts of ideal body weight for height may not be an ideal indicator of the patient's nutritional status, as apparent normal weight can mask severe muscle wasting.

Additional learning point

Body mass index (BMI) is calculated as weight in kilograms divided by height in metres squared. Normal BMI is in the range 20–25kg/m^2; BMI in the range 14–15kg/m^2 is associated with significant mortality.

Other measures of nutritional status include creatinine/height index, absolute lymphocyte count (but this may be affected by malignancy, chemotherapy, zinc deficiency, age and non-specific stress), hypocholesterolaemia, tests of muscle function such as grip strength, and respiratory muscle function analysis. The use of biochemical markers in the acute postoperative phase to assess nutritional status is not recommended. Tools such as the Malnutrition Universal Screening Tool (British Association for Parenteral and Enteral Nutrition [BAPEN], 2003) shown in *Figure 7.1* can be used within 24 hours of admission and quickly identify those at nutritional risk or suffering from malnutrition. Historically, however, their use has been variable, dependent on user uptake, and their effectiveness may thus be undermined (Kennedy, 2000).

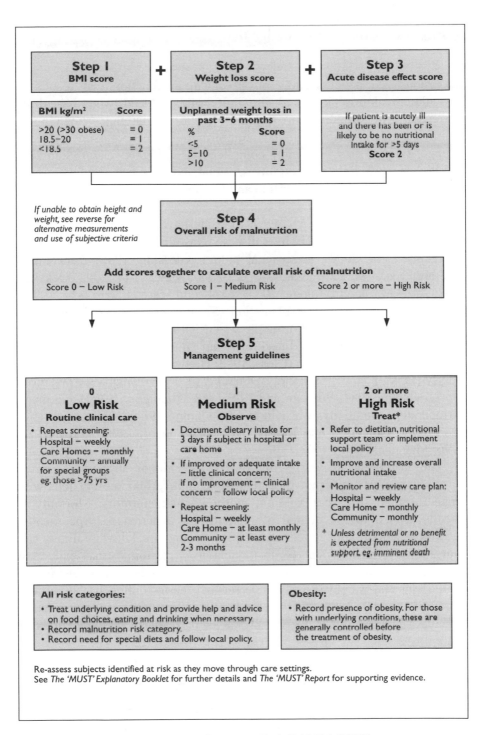

Figure 7.1: Malnutrition Universal Screening Tool (BAPEN, 2003)

The role of nutrition in health

Undernourished patients show physiological dysfunction that results in muscular weakness, impaired immunity and reduced wound healing. Compared with normally nourished patients with similar underlying clinical problems, undernourished patients require more intensive nursing and have a longer hospital stay with more complications, a higher readmission rate, and higher morbidity and mortality, especially from sepsis (Walesby *et al*, 1979; Weinsier *et al*, 1979; Warnold and Lundholm, 1984; Windsor and Hill, 1988; Stott, 2000).

Prospective randomised controlled trials have shown that nutritional support improves outcome in liver disease (Nasrallah and Gallambos, 1980; Mangiante *et al*, 2002), acute renal failure (Glessing, 1986), pancreatitis (Kalfarentzos *et al*, 1997; Eatock *et al*, 2000; Meier *et al*, 2002, Ockenga *et al*, 2002; Marik and Zaloga, 2004), Crohn's disease (Lochs *et al*, 1991), bone marrow and liver transplantation (Szeluga *et al*, 1987; Weisdorf *et al*, 1987; Mehta *et al*, 1995), emphysema/COPD (Efthimiou *et al*, 1988; Rogers *et al*, 1992), fractured neck of femur (Bastow *et al*, 1983; Delmi *et al*, 1990), pressure ulceration (Closs, 1993; Houwing *et al*, 2003), care of the elderly (Larsson *et al*, 1990; Gray-Donald *et al*, 1995), pregnancy (Warnold and Lundholm, 1984; Windsor and Hill, 1988; Allen *et al*, 1994) and many perioperative conditions (Warnold and Lundholm, 1984; Windsor and Hill, 1988; Beier-Holgersen and Boesby, 1996; Carr *et al*, 1996; Kudsk *et al*, 1996; Mangiante *et al*, 2002).

The instigation of early, appropriate nutritional support is aimed at avoidance of undernutrition-related complications associated with longer hospital stay, re-admission, morbidity and mortality. Mortality is directly related to the degree of malnutrition experienced. Specifically, nutritional support aims to reduce infection, wound breakdown, fatigue, and neurological, psychological, cardiac, respiratory, gastrointestinal, endocrine and functional impairment. Impaired appetite, grossly inadequate intake of nutrients and weight loss continue for long periods after discharge; it is therefore important for the ward nurse to identify patients who are not eating or have a reduced intake before discharge, particularly during periods of acute illness.

Additional learning point
Patients with poor nutritional status suffer many problems, and recovery time may be increased.

Nutritional care should be directed towards meeting the patient's physiological and psychosocial needs. Many of the problems surrounding the safe, timely, effective delivery of adequate nutrition for acutely ill patients can be overcome by a committed, multidisciplinary nutrition team.

The main factors contributing to poor nutritional management of patients are poor nutritional assessment strategies, poor medical and nursing knowledge and practice and inadequate facilities. Many iatrogenic reasons for non-establishment of feeding have been suggested, including discontinuation of feed for 'head-down' procedures, non-availability of feed, abdominal distension, diarrhoea and vomiting. Problems with nasogastric tube insertion or correct placement can also delay the commencement of feeding. This may result in patients receiving low volumes of prescribed enteral feed and may include periods of up to 6 days without nutritional support (Medley *et al*, 1993; Iapichino *et al*, 2004).

Treatments and interventions

It is important that all patients are fed. For those who are able to absorb adequate amounts of nutrients, fluids and electrolytes via the gastrointestinal tract, enteral feeding should be used. While patients should be encouraged to eat normally, this is rarely viable for those who are acutely ill. Patients who cannot eat normally may receive nutritional support by either the enteral or parenteral route.

Enteral nutrition

In enteral nutrition, nutrients are delivered to the gastrointestinal tract distal to the oral cavity via a tube, catheter or stoma. Enteral nutrition takes advantage of the stomach's natural function of adjusting osmolarity, mixing and serving as a reservoir. It ensures that nutrients are given the maximal amount of time for absorption. Enteral nutrition stimulates normal gut function and maintains gut integrity, cilia height and maximum absorptive effect of the gut.

Additional learning point

The use of enteral feed is cost-effective and should be the method of choice where the gut is working but oral intake is inadequate.

Early postoperative enteral feeding is a valid alternative to parenteral feeding in patients undergoing major surgery. Immediate postoperative enteral feeding in patients undergoing intestinal resection is safe (Bengmark *et al*, 2001), prevents an increase in gut mucosal permeability and produces a positive nitrogen balance. Feeding within 6 hours of insult can improve the hormonal response to stress, improve wound healing and decrease the incidence of bowel obstruction and septic complications.

Various nutritional parameters can be returned to normal more quickly with the use of enteral nutrition than with parenteral nutrition. Patients who receive early enteral feeding demonstrate significant reductions in the incidence of anastomotic dehiscence, wound infection, sepsis, pneumonia, intra-abdominal abscess and mortality (Lewis *et al*, 2001).

There are several methods of enteral feeding that can be considered, including:

- Nasogastric feeeding
- Nasojejunal feeding
- Percutaneous endoscopic gastrostomy (PEG).

If the patient has a gastrointestinal tract that is capable of absorbing adequate fluids and nutrients to maintain health and hydration but is unable to eat normally, feeding via a nasogastric tube is the preferred route of feed delivery for short-term use, provided that there are no problems with delayed gastric emptying or pulmonary aspiration.

Placement of a nasogastric tube

Nasogastric feeding entails passing a fine-bore feeding tube into the patient's stomach via the nose to deliver feed. This may be done under direct vision using a laryngoscope by experienced and qualified personnel, or by passage of the tube without direct vision. Although these tubes can also be passed via the mouth, there is a risk of the patient biting the tube.

> **Additional learning point**
> Prior to insertion of a nasogastric tube, the procedure should be explained to the patient, and the patient's verbal informed consent sought (if possible).

Positioning the patient in a semi-recumbent position may help passage of the tube by gravity. Measurement of the tube should be done before attempting to pass the tube. The tube should be measured from the tip of the nose to the tip of the ear to the xiphisternum and a corresponding mark on the tube made. For an average adult patient, this will mean approximately 50–55cm at the nostril. The tube should be advanced slowly towards the back of the throat through a cleared nostril. The lubricant used should be water as opposed to a water-soluble lubricant, as the latter may potentially block the tube or affect the pH of any aspirate obtained once the tube is in place. If the tube fails to advance or the patient complains of severe ear pain or shows signs of respiratory distress (tachypnoea, cyanosis, oxygen desaturation), the procedure should be stopped as this may indicate misplacement of the tube.

Inadvertent tube removal is the most common reason for removing the tube. The tube is traditionally secured with a hypoallergenic fixative device at the patient's nostril and then secured to the patient's cheek. A technique for the use of a nasal bridle has been described, but should be used with caution for confused patients because of the risk of inadvertent trauma to the nares and septum.

Nasogastric tubes are made from polyvinyl chloride (PVC), latex, polyurethane or silicone. Polyurethane is superior to silicone in reducing clogging of feed. The tube wall of a polyurethane tube may be thinner, allowing higher flow rates for the same external diameter. PVC tubes can become brittle if left in situ for too long (>10 days) and may be damaged by radiotherapy.

Problems associated with tube placement

There are many possible problems associated with nasogastric tube insertion, and competence in placing a nasogastric tube is a skill that nurses develop. Ensure that you check local policy related to achieving competence in tube placement and checking correct positioning of the tube. Potential problems include:

* Rhinitis
* Pharyngitis

- Oesophagitis
- Oesophageal erosion
- Stricture
- Perforation
- Upper gastrointestinal tract bleeding
- Intracranial penetration
- Tracheobronchial intubation (risk 0.9–2.4%)
- Tracheopleural intubation through intact artificial airways
- Pneumothorax
- Coiling of the tube in the mouth, either in front of the teeth or under the tongue, causing it to fail to advance.

Checking nasogastric tube placement

Once the nasogastric tube has advanced to the required length, its position should be checked by aspirating gastric residual and testing its pH with indicator paper. If the pH test paper shows an acidic reaction with a pH of ≤5.5 (National Patient Safety Agency [NPSA], 2005) it is safe to use the tube for the administration of feed, fluid or medication. This procedure should be repeated each time the tube is used for any of these purposes, although repeat aspirations may increase the risk of tube blockage. Failure to check tube placement may result in pulmonary aspiration going unnoticed and an adverse outcome.

Additional learning point
Nasogastric tube position should be checked before starting feed, after feed has been stopped for bag changes or rest, and if there is any possibility of tube dislodgement. pH paper must be used to test the gastric aspirate and a pH of ≤5.5 obtained before feed is restarted (NPSA, 2005).

Checking the position of the tube by auscultation is unsafe because of the risk of hearing transmitted bowel sounds, and may only be 60% reliable. Testing gastric aspirate with litmus paper is also unsafe as bronchial secretions may turn blue litmus paper pink, and should not be used.

The nurse should note that the administration of prokinetic agents can affect the ability to obtain gastric aspirate, because of their effect in increasing stomach emptying. Ninety-five per cent of nurses report checking gastric aspirate 4-hourly and 50% discard the aspirates (Mateo, 1996). Also, patients receiving antacids, H2 antagonists or proton pump inhibitors may have an unusually high gastric pH. Aspiration tests on these patients may therefore not be accurate, and it may be necessary to repeat the aspirate test to avoid the time around drug administration. In patients for whom an aspirate is unobtainable, or who have an aspirate with a pH >5.5, chest X-ray may be necessary to confirm the correct positioning of the nasogastric tube. It must be borne in mind that the X-ray is only conclusive at the time it is taken, as the tube may move with vomiting, retching, coughing, pulling or patient movement.

Problems arising from poor gastric absorption

Following illness, trauma or surgery, gastroparesis and colonoparesis inhibit the absorption of enteral feeds delivered to the stomach. High gastric residual volumes occur in about 35% of patients who are acutely ill, leading to an increased risk of gastro-oesophageal reflux and pulmonary aspiration. Erythromycin and metoclopramide have been shown to be beneficial in promoting gastric emptying and allowing continuation of enteral feeds; if it is not possible to feed the patient via the nasogastric route, other options can be considered.

Nasojejunal feeding

Studies have demonstrated that small bowel function remains within the normal range or only slightly depressed during illness, trauma or surgery (Bengmark *et al*, 2001). The instigation of nasojejunal feeding may be considered if gastric emptying is not occurring. This route takes advantage of the functional small bowel and its ability to absorb nutrients and fluids, avoiding the need for parenteral nutrition. The absence of bowel sounds should not preclude the commencement of enteral feeding.

Additional indications for nasojejunal feeding include hyperemesis gravidarum, acute pancreatitis, postoperative paralytic ileus, obstructive lesions high in the gastrointestinal tract, partial gastric outlet obstruction, gastric or duodenal fistula, high risk of pulmonary aspiration, chemotherapy-induced nausea and severe mucositis.

Nasojejunal tube insertion is generally undertaken by medical staff, and additional caution is exercised in patients with:

* Maxillo-facial disorders or surgery
* Post-laryngectomy

- Oropharyngeal tumours
- Post-oropharyngeal surgery
- Prolonged clotting times
- Suspected or actual skull fractures
- Unstable cervical spine injuries involving C4 or above.

Nasojejunal tube placement

Nasojejunal feeding tubes may be inserted in two main ways:

- Endoscopically at the bedside of the critically ill patient by appropriately skilled endoscopy staff
- Using a coiled-tip tube not under direct vision, by experienced staff, with peristalsis advancing the tube to the jejunum in a mean of 7.6 hours (Mangiante *et al*, 2000).

The patient should be monitored throughout the endoscopic procedure using a pulse oximeter and cardiac monitor, and the readings recorded, as sedation may be administered during the procedure to facilitate placement. Emergency equipment, including oxygen, suction and a resuscitation trolley, should be nearby, with adequate staff skilled in resuscitative procedures available if needed.

An X-ray request form for abdominal radiography should be completed post-insertion. This X-ray should be completed and reviewed by a registrar or consultant and the result of the review documented in the medical notes before using the tube for feed or drug administration.

Factors that increase the chance of successful tube insertion distal to the pylorus include air insufflation and the use of unweighted-end tubes, as these pass more successfully than those with a weighted end. The nurse should observe the patient for tube blockage, tube dislodgement and septal or oesophageal erosion, intestinal perforation, small bowel necrosis (Lawlor *et al*, 1998) and bleeding in the jejunum.

Percutaneous endoscopic gastrostomy (PEG)

Gastrostomy may be considered for the acutely ill patient with a functional gastrointestinal tract who is likely to require long-term nutritional support (>6 weeks). Gastrostomy feeding takes advantage of the stomach's natural function of adjusting osmolarity, mixing and serving as a reservoir. It ensures that nutrients are given the maximal time for absorption, eliminating the risk of oesophageal or nasal mucosal injury. Feeding can usually recommence within 24 hours.

Complications of PEG feeding

Approximately 9% of patients receiving PEG feeding develop complications. These include:

- Aspiration pneumonia
- Subcutaneous abscess
- Gastric perforation
- Gastric haemorrhage
- Gastro-colic fistula
- Wound dehiscence
- Tube blockage/malfunction, tube dislodgement
- Increased peristomal infection rate
- Cellulitis
- Peritonitis.

Nursing care of the PEG tube

Routine care of the PEG tube should include:

- Observation of the insertion site for signs of local infection, ie. redness, tenderness, swelling, exudates and heat. If these are present in conjunction with pyrexia of unknown origin, the site should be swabbed and the swab sent to the microbiology department. Additionally, a short course of antibiotics (orally if tolerated by the patient or via the PEG tube) may be considered.

- Care of the fixation plate on the outside of the PEG tube. The fixation plate should be next to the patient's skin at all times; if it not positioned correctly, the 'stoma' will not form, increasing the risk of peritonitis. Within one week of insertion of the PEG tube, consideration should be given to daily rotation of the tube in the stoma being formed between the patient's abdominal wall and the inner stomach wall; this will facilitate formation of the stoma and avoid buried bumper syndrome.

- Monitoring for tube blockage is important as enteral feeding tubes block easily in 6–10% of cases. This may be related to the administration of elixirs or crushed medications via the tube, poor flushing of the tube, or commonly the precipitation of protein feed in the tube. Nurses administering medications via PEG tubes should flush the PEG with 20ml of sterile water, or whatever is recommended by local policy, after each drug is given. The best method of unblocking a nasoenteric tube is flushing with water (Haynes-Johnson, 1986) using a large-bore syringe with a minimum of 20ml of water.

Administration of enteral feeds

When correct positioning of the PEG tube has been confirmed, use of the tube for gastric aspiration or the administration of feed or medications may commence. Isonitrogenous sterile feed (1 kcal/ml) is used for the majority of patients receiving enteral nutrition. The patient should be nursed in a semi-recumbent position to reduce the risk of pulmonary aspiration. Once the administration of feed is commenced, usually via a rate-controlled pump, it is common and good practice to check the flow rate within one hour of commencement of feed in order to avoid inadvertent over-infusion.

There is traditionally a minimum 4-hour break in feed infusion every 24 hours. However, in critical care areas it is becoming common to administer feed over a 24-hour period to facilitate tight glycaemic control, which has demonstrated improved patient outcomes (VanDen Berghe *et al*, 2001). The break in feed infusion allows the gastric pH to become more acidic, thereby avoiding bacterial overgrowth, which may spread to the respiratory system via the oesophagus and trachea. Before recommencing feeding, aspiration is performed to check the gastric pH and ensure correct placement of the tube, and to assess gastric residual volume in the gut as this is traditionally used to measure tolerance of nasogastric enteral feeding.

Bacterial contamination of enteral feeds is cumulative and common. It is related to the many manipulations of the feed and feeding system, preparation of the feed and its administration. The use of tap water rather than sterile water in the reconstitution of feeds and flushing of enteral feeding tubes, the re-use of enteral feed containers and the repeated aspiration of gastric residual via the tube all increase the risk of contamination. The design of the feed administration set and duration of use may also be significant factors. Care should be taken to use a clean technique in the handling of feeds and infusion lines: handwashing, the use of non-sterile gloves and an apron are appropriate.

Parenteral nutrition

Patients with acute or chronic intestinal failure due to reduced intestinal absorption require macronutrient and/or water and electrolyte supplements to maintain health and/or growth (Nightingale, 2001). In such patients, enteral nutrition, in addition to the administration of intravenous electrolytes and fluids, may be considered. If these interventions are insufficient or contraindicated by the patient's condition, parenteral nutrition is the method of nutritional support. This consists of the administration of an amino-acid based solution directly into a large vein; the main constituents of the regimen are water, protein, carbohydrate, fat, electrolytes, trace elements and vitamins. Parenteral nutrition usage is common in acutely ill patients. Parenteral nutrition is delivered through a large central vein in most situations; peripheral parenteral nutrition is possible, but is associated with an increased risk of extravasation, thrombophlebitis and abscess formation at the administration site, making it a high-risk procedure.

Line placement for parenteral nutrition

The main veins used for central venous access are the internal and external jugular veins, right and left subclavian veins, and the cephalic and basilic veins. The femoral veins are occasionally used, although this route is thought to be associated with a higher risk of infection.

Use of the internal jugular vein is associated with several problems, including catheter occlusion and irritation due to head movement and difficulty in maintaining an intact dressing. The external jugular vein is more easily observable, but it varies in size and the junction with the subclavian vein makes cannulation difficult.

The subclavian vein is the vein of choice for long-term central venous access for parenteral nutrition. The subclavian vein is often used because it requires the shortest length of catheter, it has a rapid blood flow due to its size, and there is less risk of irritation and obstruction. The central venous access device is easily secured to the chest wall. Contraindications to the use of the subclavian vein include superior vena cava obstruction, irradiation of the chest, clavicular fracture and malignancy of the neck. Pneumothorax is the most common complication of this route.

The basilic and cephalic veins may be used for the insertion of peripherally inserted central catheters [PICCs]. Although the basilic and cephalic veins have a smaller diameter than the subclavian or jugular veins, cannulation at the inner aspect of the elbow allows easy advancement of a PICC to the junction of the superior vena cava and the right atrium. Also, PICCs have lower complication rates than chest- or neck-inserted lines, with a significant reduction in the risk of pneumothorax, haemorrhage and catheter-related sepsis.

A significant factor in the common use of PICCs is ease of insertion. Placement of parenteral nutrition lines in the subclavian or jugular veins requires the patient to be laid flat with head inverted for part of the procedure. This allows venous engorgement of the vein to be cannulated, making visualisation easier for the inserter. Insertion of a PICC does not require the same positioning of the patient, and this may increase tolerance of the procedure by patients with compromised cardiac and respiratory function. Insertion of all types of central lines should be undertaken with at least local anaesthesia, using full barrier precautions and a chlorhexidine-based skin-cleansing agent. Insertion-related complications of central venous access devices occur in 3–12% of patients and correlate directly with the experience of the inserter (Mughal, 1989).

All lines except PICCs are usually sutured in place; sterile adhesive strips such as Steristrips™ may be used to secure the lines. The lines are then covered by an adhesive sterile dressing. A sterile, gauze-based dressing is commonly used for PICCs and a transparent film dressing for neck lines, but the nurse should check local policy. Dressings need to allow easy inspection of the catheter entry site for localised infection. However, it should be borne in mind that the catheter position may inadvertently be altered when changing this dressing unless care is observed. Additionally, there is a risk of fluid pooling at the catheter entry site from seepage of sweat or blood down the catheter; this fluid may collect under the dressing and become infected.

As with any central vein access line, a chest X-ray must always be taken and reviewed before using the line for infusion. The purpose of the X-ray is to confirm correct positioning of the line and to check for pneumothorax. The tip of the parenteral nutrition catheter should lie at the junction of the superior vena cava and right atrium. If the tip of the line lies in the axillary vein or the median segment of the subclavian vein, there is an increased risk of thrombosis and venous occlusion. If the X-ray indicates pneumothorax, an intercostal chest drain may be required if respiratory function is compromised. Insertion of a chest drain must be undertaken by appropriately qualified and experienced medical staff. Early signs of pneumothorax may include tachypnoea, dyspnoea, tachycardia, hypoxia with potential confusion and reduced air entry on the affected side. Careful observation of the patient for the first 6 hours post-insertion of the line is vital.

Risks associated with parental feeding lines

Complications occur in 25% of parenteral nutrition episodes. Parenteral nutrition line-related sepsis is a common reason for cessation of parenteral nutrition. Parenteral nutrition is associated with a significant level of morbidity through catheter related sepsis and metabolic and mechanical problems, which are potentially life threatening. The risk of catheter colonisation is around 25% and the risk of infection around 5% (Adal and Farr, 1996; Maki *et al*, 1997) in lines that are well managed; the risk of infection may rise to 70% in lines where staff knowledge of line and infusion care is poor (Kennedy *et al*, 2001). While the majority of complications are infective, requiring removal of the central venous catheter, many episodes of catheter-related sepsis may be iatrogenic, with healthcare staff not being aware of care needs. Bedside tests are being developed for the detection of catheter-related sepsis, which obviate catheter removal and provide a cost-effective means of managing patients with suspected catheter-related sepsis.

Additional learning point
The key to reducing the risk of infection in a parenteral nutrition line is adequate training and maintenance of competency of medical and nursing staff (Kennedy *et al*, 2002).

Risk factors for line sepsis may include:

* The use of multi-lumen lines as opposed to dedicated single-lumen lines
* The material from which the line is constructed
* Increased number of connections between the parenteral nutrition administration set and the patient's central venous access device
* Increased number of manipulations of the line
* Subcutaneous tunnelling of the line at insertion may prolong catheter life but have equivocal benefit in the management of catheter-related sepsis.

Managing a potentially infected line

Infection of a parenteral nutrition line is currently confirmed by culture of blood samples from the feeding line and from a peripheral vein, using strict aseptic technique for the collection of samples to reduce the risk of cross-contamination. Exclusion of other sources of infection, by culture of a wound swab from the parenteral nutrition line entry site, sputum, endotracheal aspirate, urine, wound swabs, drain exudates and stool, should also be considered.

Additional learning point
It is important to ascertain the source of sepsis before interrupting a patient's parenteral nutrition. The decision to remove a parenteral nutrition line because of suspected infection should be a multidisciplinary one.

The most common organism cultured in approximately 70% of line infections is a coagulase-negative staphylococcus (Staphylococcus epidermidis). Characteristically in the case of a line infection, this will colonise the inner lumen of the line. Once the parenteral nutrition infusion is commenced, if the line is infected one would expect to see a spike in temperature within one hour of commencement of the feed. At this point, the nurse should stop the feed, inform medical staff and commence regular formal observation of the patient. If the parenteral nutrition line is the precipitant of the symptoms of infection, the temperature will have settled within one hour. If this is the case, discontinue the parenteral nutrition, flush the line with prescribed 0.9% sodium chloride and inform the nutrition team. If the temperature remains elevated it is likely that there is another primary source of infection causing the pyrexia and the parenteral nutrition can be recommenced (*Figure 7.2*).

Complications of parental nutrition

Apart from the risk of sepsis discussed above, there are other possible complications of parenteral nutrition. Feeding should therefore only be administered by this route when the risks have been considered alongside the benefits. Enteral feeding is always first choice. Potential complications of parenteral nutrition include:

- Catheter occlusion or dislodgement
- Hyperglycaemia
- Rebound hypoglycaemia

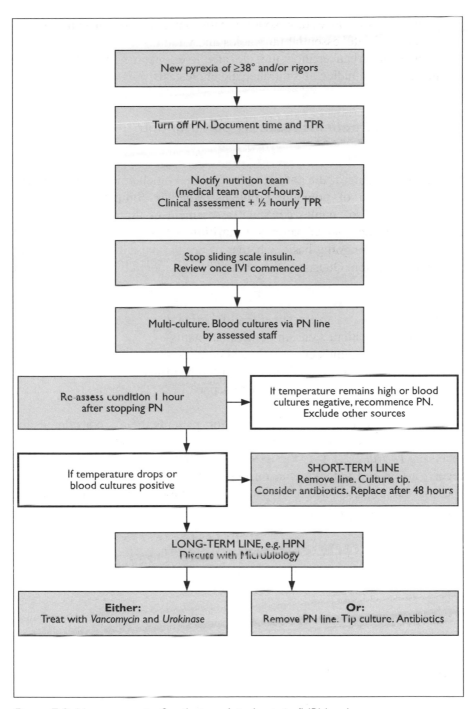

Figure 7.2: Management of catheter-related sepsis (HPN = home parenteral nutrition; PN = parenteral nutrition; TPR = temperature, pulse and respiratory rate)

- Deficiencies of potassium, sodium, phosphate, zinc, magnesium, trace elements, folate, essential fatty acids and vitamins
- Hepatic disturbances including elevated liver enzymes, fatty infiltration, jaundice and intrahepatic cholestasis.

Monitoring of patients receiving parental nutrition

Routine monitoring of the patient's physical and biochemical status ensures early recognition of potential problems, whether clinical, metabolic or mechanical. It also enables continual assessment of the patient's progress to ensure that the goal of parenteral nutrition is being met. It is important to assess, on an ongoing basis, whether or not the patient requires ongoing parenteral nutrition. Questions that should be considered by the clinical team include:

- Is the patient's gastrointestinal tract functional?
- What is the patient's current nutritional status?
- What is the patient's current clinical condition?
- Is the patient's nutritional status likely to be affected by any (proposed) treatment, investigation or ongoing sepsis?

Regular blood tests are required for patients being considered for parenteral nutrition, and as part of ongoing assessment while they are receiving it. *Table 7.1* lists the tests recommended for patients before they receive parenteral nutrition and during the time they are receiving it. The specific nursing care needs of patients receiving parenteral nutrition are summarised in *Appendix 7*.

Table 7.1: Monitoring of patients receiving parenteral nutrition

Before starting parenteral nutrition

Blood	U&Es	Glucose
	LFTs	Calcium and phosphate
	Magnesium	FBC
	INR	Clotting screen
	Zinc and copper	Folate and vitamin B_{12}
	Triglycerides	Cholesterol

Daily if patient is unstable or new

Blood	U&Es	LFTs
	Calcium and phosphate	FBC
	Glucose	

In first week of parenteral nutrition

24-hour urine	Electrolytes	Urea
	Creatinine	

Twice weekly if patient is stable

Blood	U&Es	LFTs
	Calcium and phosphate	FBC
Random urine sodium	Twice weekly	

Weekly

Blood	FBC	Clotting screen
	Trace elements (eg. copper, zinc, selenium)	
	Folate and vitamin B_{12}	

Fortnightly

24-hour urine	Electrolytes	Urea and creatinine

FBC = full blood count; INR = International normalised ratio; LFTs = liver function tests; U&Es = urea and electrolytes

Key learning points for *Chapter 7*

- Early appropriate nutritional support improves the outcome in patients who are acutely ill. Nurses work as part of a multidisciplinary team in the safe and effective assessment and management of nutritional input. Various enteral feeding options are available; these should be explored for all patients in the first instance. The option of parenteral nutrition is effective, but is associated with potentially serious complications that need to be managed by experienced and trained staff.

- Adequate nutrition is necessary to ensure survival, growth and repair of tissues and cells.

- Undernourished patients show physiological dysfunction that results in muscle weakness, impaired immunity and reduced wound healing.

- Avoidance of undernourishment is important, particularly in acutely ill patients.

- Patient assessment should include the ability to eat and drink, gut function and functional ability. Optimisation of nutritional input can then be achieved.

- Enteral or parenteral nutrition can be given, but enteral nutrition is always first choice.

- Before using a nasogastric tube to administer medications, fluids or feed, the nurse must confirm the correct positioning of the tube. Remember to check the placement of nasogastric tubes using pH paper on an aspirate of the gastric residual; pH should be <5.5.

- Monitor for early signs of sepsis in patients with parenteral nutrition lines in situ.

- Adherence to strict aseptic technique will ensure reduction of infection risks in all patients, but particularly in parenteral nutrition lines.

Revision questions – nutrition

1. Why is nutrition important?
2. When should the acutely ill patient be fed?
3. Why is it important to ascertain the position of a nasogastric tube before use, and how can the position of the tube be determined accurately?
4. Is auscultation an effective method of checking nasogastric tube position?
5. What are the indications for PEG placement?
6. What complications may arise from PEG placement?
7. What are the indications for parenteral nutrition?
8. What are the complications associated with parenteral nutrition line insertion and administration?
9. What are the risk factors for parenteral nutrition-related line sepsis?
10. What monitoring is required for patients receiving parenteral nutrition?

Answers on page 199

References

Adal KA, Farr BM (1996) Central venous catheter-related infections: a review. *Nutrition* **12**: 208–213

Allen LH, Lung'aho MS, Shaheen M *et al* (1994) Maternal body mass index and pregnancy outcome in the Nutrition Collaborative Research Support Program. *European Journal of Clinical Nutrition* **48**(Suppl 3): S68–S76

Bastow MD, Rawlings J, Allison SP (1983) Benefits of supplementary tube feeding after fractured neck of femur: a randomised controlled trial. *British Medical Journal* **287**: 1589–1592

Beier-Holgersen R, Boesby S (1996) Influence of post-operative enteral nutrition on post-surgical infections. *Gut* **39**: 833–835

British Association for Parenteral and Enteral Nutrition (2003) Malnutrition Universal Screening Tool. Available at: http://www.bapen.org.uk/the-must.htm (last accessed 18.01.06)

Bengmark S, Andersson R, Mangiante G (2001) Uninterrupted perioperative enteral nutrition. *Clinical Nutrition* **20**(1): 11–19

Carr CS, Ling KDE, Boulos P, Singer M (1996) Randomised trials of safety and efficacy of immediate postoperative enteral feeding in patients undergoing gastrointestinal resection. *British Medical Journal* **312**(7035): 869–871

Closs SJ (1993) Orthopaedics. Malnutrition: the key to pressure sores? *Nursing Standard* **8**(4): 32–36

Delmi M, Rapin CH, Bengoa JM *et al* (1990) Dietary supplementation in elderly patients with fractured neck of femur. *Lancet* **335**: 1013–1016

Eatock FC, Brombacher GD, Steven A *et al* (2000) Nasogastric feeding in severe acute pancreatitis may be practical and safe. *International Journal of Pancreatology* **28**(1): 25–31

Efthimiou J, Fleming J, Gomes C, Spiro SG (1988) The effect of supplementary oral nutrition in poorly nourished patients with chronic obstructive pulmonary disease. *American Review of Respiratory Disease* **137**: 1075–1082

Glessing J (1986) Addition of amino acids to peritoneal dialysis fluid. *Lancet* **ii**: 812

Gray-Donald K, Payette H, Boutier V (1995) Randomized clinical trial of nutritional supplementation shows little effect on functional status among free-living frail elderly. *Journal of Nutrition* **125**: 2965–2971

Haynes-Johnson V (1986) Tube feeding complications: causes, prevention and therapy. *Nutritional Support Services* **6**(3): 17–22

Heyland DK, Schroter-Noppe D, Drover JW *et al* (2003) Nutrition support in the critical care setting: current practice in Canadian ICUs – opportunities for improvement? *Journal of Parenteral and Enteral Nutrition* **27**(1): 74–83

Houwing RH, Rozendaal M, Wouters-Wesseling W *et al* (2003) A randomised, double-blind assessment of the effect of nutritional supplementation on the prevention of pressure ulcers in hip-fracture patients. *Clinical Nutrition* **22**(4): 401–406

Iapichino G, Rossi C, Radrizzani D *et al*, for the GiViTi (Italian group for the evaluation of interventions in intensive care medicine) (2004) Nutrition given to critically ill during high level/complex care (on Italian ICUs). *Clinical Nutrition* **23**: 409–416

Kalfarentzos F, Kehagias J, Mead N *et al* (1997) Early enteral nutrition is superior to parenteral nutrition in severe acute pancreatitis: results of a randomized prospective trial. *British Journal of Surgery* **84**: 1665–1669

Kennedy JF (2000) Quality in nutritional assessment: the role of the nutrition nurse in the implementation of a nutritional assessment tool. *Proceedings of the Nutrition Society* **59**

Kennedy JF, Nightingale JMD, Currie M (2001) Quality benefits of a nutrition team. *Clinical Nutrition* **20**(Suppl 3): 70

Kennedy JF, Nightingale JMD, Baker ML (2002) Nurse training is the key factor in reducing catheter-related sepsis rates in patients receiving parenteral nutrition. *Clinical Nutrition* **21**(Suppl 1): 73

Kudsk KA, Minard G, Croce MA *et al* (1996) A randomised trial of isonitrogenous enteral diets after severe trauma. An immune-enhancing diet reduces septic complications. *Annals of Surgery* **224**: 531–543

Larsson J, Unosoon M, Ek A-C *et al* (1990) Effect of dietary supplementation on nutritional status and clinical outcome in 501 geriatric patients – a randomised study. *Clinical Nutrition* **9**: 179–184

Lawlor DK, Inculet RI, Malthaner RA (1998) Small bowel necrosis associated with jejunal tube feeding. *Canadian Journal of Surgery* **41**(6): 459–462

Lewis SJ, Egger M, Sylvester PA, Thomas S (2001) Early enteral feeding versus 'nil by mouth' after gastrointestinal surgery: a systematic review and meta-analysis of controlled trials. *British Medical Journal* **323**(7316): 773–776

Lochs H, Steinhardt HJ, Klaus-Wentz B *et al* (1991) Comparison of enteral nutrition and drug treatment in active Crohn's disease. *Gastroenterology* **101**: 881–888

Maki DG, Stolz SM, Wheeler S, Mermel LA (1997) Prevention of central venous catheter-related bloodstream infection by use of an antiseptic-impregnated catheter. A randomised, controlled trial. *Annals of Internal Medicine* **127**: 257–266

Mangiante G, Marini P, Fratucello GB *et al* (2000) The Bengmark tube in surgical practice and in the critically ill patient. *Chirurgia Italiana* **52**(5): 573–578

Mangiante G, Rossi L, Carluccio S *et al* (2002) Influence of enteral nutrition on cytokine response in resective liver surgery. *Chirurgia Italiana* **54**(5): 613–619

Marik PE, Zaloga GP (2004) Meta-analysis of parenteral nutrition versus enteral nutrition in patients with acute pancreatitis. *British Medical Journal* doi: 10.1136/bmj.38118.593900.55.

Mateo MA (1996) Nursing management of enteral tube feedings. *Heart & Lung* **25**(4): 318–323

McWhirter J, Pennington CR (1994) Incidence of malnutrition in hospital. *British Medical Journal* **308**: 945–948

Medley F, Stechmiller J, Field A (1993) Complications of enteral nutrition in hospitalised patients with artificial airways. *Clinical Nursing Research* **2**(2): 212–223

Mehta PL, Alaka KJ, Filo RS *et al* (1995) Nutrition support following liver transplantation: comparison of jejunal versus parenteral routes. *Clinical Transplantation* **9**(5): 364–369

Meier R, Beglinger C, Layer P *et al*; ESPEN Consensus Group (2002) ESPEN guidelines on nutrition in acute pancreatitis. *Clinical Nutrition* **21**(2):173–183

Mughal MM (1989) Complications of intravenous feeding catheters. *British Journal of Surgery* **76**: 15–21

Nasrallah SM, Galambos JT (1980) Amino acid therapy of alcoholic hepatitis. *Lancet* **ii**: 1276–1277

National Patient Safety Agency (NPSA) (2005) How to confirm the correct position of nasogastric feeding tubes in infants, children and adults. Available at: http://www.npsa.nhs.uk/site/media/documents/857_Insert-finalWeb.pdf (last accessed 17.01.06)

Nightingale JMD (2001) Definition and classification of intestinal failure. In: Nightingale JMD (Ed) *Intestinal Failure*. Greenwich Medical Media, London

Ockenga J, Borchert K, Rifai K *et al* (2002) Effect of glutamine-enriched total parenteral nutrition in patients with acute severe pancreatitis. *Clinical Nutrition* **21**(5): 409–416

Rogers RM, Donahoe M, Constantino J (1992) Physiologic effects of oral supplemental feeding in malnourished patients with chronic obstructive pulmonary disease. A randomized control study. *American Review of Respiratory Disease* **146**(6): 1511–1517

Stott S (2000) Recent advances in intensive care. *British Medical Journal* **320**: 358–361

Szeluga DJ, Stuart RK, Brookmeyer R *et al* (1987) Nutritional support of bone marrow transplant recipients: a prospective, randomized clinical trial comparing total parenteral nutrition to an enteral feeding program. *Cancer Research* **47**(12): 3309–3316

VanDen Berghe G, Wouters P, Weekers F *et al* (2001) Intensive insulin therapy in critically ill patients. *New England Journal of Medicine* **345**(19): 1359–1367

Walesby RK, Goode AW, Spink TJ *et al* (1979) Nutritional status of patients requiring cardiac surgery. *Journal of Thoracic and Cardiovascular Surgery* **77**: 570–576

Warnold I, Lundholm K (1984) Clinical significance of pre-operative nutritional status in 215 non-cancer patients. *Annals of Surgery* **199**: 299–305

Weinsier RL, Hunker EM, Krumdieck CL, Butterworth CE (1979) A prospective evaluation of general medical patients during the course of hospitalisation. *American Journal of Clinical Nutrition* **32**: 418–426

Weisdorf SA, Lysne J, Wind D *et al* (1987) Positive effect of prophylactic total parenteral nutrition on long-term outcome of bone marrow transplantation. *Transplantation* **43**(6): 833–838

Windsor JA, Hill GL (1988) Weight loss with physiological impairment: a basic indicator for surgical risk. *Annals of Surgery* **207**: 290–296

CHAPTER 8

Pain management

S Daykin

Assessment and observations

History

When taking a history of pain from a patient, it is important to consider the following:

- How long has the patient had the pain?
- Where is the pain situated?
- What type of pain does the patient have (neuropathic or visceral)?
- What makes the pain worse?
- What makes the pain better?
- Current analgesia
- Effectiveness of analgesia
- Previous medical conditions.

Defining pain

All human beings experience pain at some time in their life – this may range from a headache to surgical intervention. Pain is a complex phenomenon that is both universal and unique. Although everyone experiences pain, no two people experience the same pain in identical situations. This is easily demonstrated by recalling two patients who have undergone the same surgical procedure and reflecting on their different pain experiences.

In the past it was considered character building to suffer pain, and admirable to be able to withstand pain; even today, some patient groups still believe this to be the case. Such patients often feel that their pain is very minor compared with that of their fellow patients. No patient should be led to believe that getting treatment for his/her pain is unimportant. Long-term pain can be both negative and destructive.

> **Additional learning point**
> No patient should be led to believe that getting treatment for his/her pain is unimportant. Pain is an emotion: the fact that the patient feels pain means that the pain is real and should be treated.

Pain assessment

When a patient tells you that he/she is in pain, it is necessary to do an accurate assessment of the pain to ascertain the exact nature of the problem. Pain assessment requires good communication between nursing staff and the patient. Assessments identify the likely cause of the pain, record the context of the pain, *eg.* after coughing, and allow the nursing and medical staff to recommend a suitable form of analgesia for a particular problem.

> **Additional learning point**
> Pain assessment is an essential part of nursing practice and should be included with the basic nursing observations (Manias *et al,* 2002).

Pain assessment is needed because it:

* Is the initial step in good pain management
* Identifies the type of analgesia needed and how well the prescribed analgesia is working
* Contributes to the total physiological recovery of the patient
* May indicate a change in the general condition of the patient.

Many factors affect the accurate assessment of pain:

The nature of the illness
* Is this episode of illness likely to resolve?
* Is there a treatment regimen involved?
* Does the patient have a palliative condition that requires palliative care?

Patient's medical condition
* Is the patient well enough to communicate?

Interpretation skills
• Each member of the ward team needs to be able to interpret the assessment tool accurately; if there are different interpretations of the tool, the assessment will not be reliable.

Nurse education on the use of the tool
• Nursing staff need to be familiar with the tool used in practice and how best to use it for their patient group, otherwise it will be used inaccurately.

Communication skills of both the nurse and the patient
• Is the patient disorientated as a result of his/her condition?
• Are there cultural barriers to overcome?
• Is the patient unable to speak English as a first language, or does he/she have a condition that reduces the ability to speak (tracheotomy or laryngectomy)?
• Does the patient have poor vision or poor hearing?

Assessment of pain in patients with cognitive impairment or those who cannot respond verbally presents additional challenges for the ward nurse (Carr, 1990). Patients who have difficulty with sight and hearing can also present a challenge for the nurse when assessing pain. Skilled assessment is therefore paramount in these situations in order to avoid frustration and suffering. Adaptation of the pain assessment tool to suit individual need, along with patience and understanding, can aid assessment. All of these challenges can be overcome with innovative pain assessment.

The choice of pain assessment tool is therefore crucial to good assessment. It needs to be simple to use, easy to understand, appropriate for the patient group, reliable and valid. The usual tool used for pain assessment is a verbal scoring scale (*Table 8.1*). This involves the nurse asking the patient about his/her pain on rest and on movement, and the nurse scoring the pain accordingly.

Table 8.1: Verbal pain-rating score

0	No pain at rest and on movement
1	No pain at rest, slight pain on movement
2	Intermittent pain at rest and moderate on movement
3	Continuous pain at rest and severe on movement

Source: Hunter (1993)

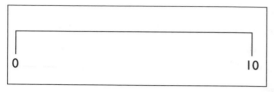

This assessment tool is good for patients who are able to communicate well with the nurse, but a patient who is acutely ill may not be able to complete this form of assessment.

Figure 8.1: Numerical ruler (visual analogue scale) used to assess pain

A pictorial assessment scale (*ie*. pictures) can be shown to patients to ascertain how they feel but they do need to have good eyesight to use this tool and many acutely ill patients may have difficulty with this. A simple numerical ruler (visual analogue scale) can also be used as a visual aid. This usually consists of a ruler marked 0 at one end and 10 at the other, where 0 = no pain and 10 = the most pain possible (*Figure 8.1*); care does need to be taken with this tool to ensure accuracy. It may be necessary to adapt your current pain assessment tool in certain situations. It is important, however, to ensure that all members of the team know which tool is being used and how to use it and interpret the scores.

Records of pain assessment are paramount. The most appropriate place to record pain assessment is on the chart used to record the patient's basic observations (blood pressure, pulse, temperature and respiratory rate). A dedicated pain assessment chart can also be used, along with any charts used for monitoring the use of patient-controlled analgesia (PCA) or epidural analgesia.

Observations

The following observations should be carried out on a patient before administering analgesia for the first time in order to obtain baseline values. This will also help the nurse to monitor any side-effects of the analgesia:

- Blood pressure
- Temperature, pulse and respiratory rate
- Pain assessment using a suitable pain assessment tool.

The following observations should then be checked following analgesia (about 30–60 minutes post-administration):

- Blood pressure
- Temperature, pulse and respiratory rate

- Pain assessment to assess the effectiveness of the analgesia
- Assessment of any nausea or itching
- Presence of side-effects: the nurse should be aware of the general side-effects of any analgesic drug administered and should always monitor the patient for their development, particularly in the first 24 hours after administration. If side-effects do occur, they should be reported to medical staff so that an alternative analgesic can be found, or medication prescribed to prevent the side-effects, such as an anti-emetic for nausea and vomiting.

If the patient is receiving epidural analgesia or PCA, other observations may be required; the nurse should check local policy regarding this practice.

Anatomy and physiology of pain

Most pain is caused by damage to tissue; damage to nerves also causes pain (neuropathic pain). But irrespective of the cause, if the patient thinks he/she is in pain, then he/she is in pain. Tissue or nerve damage can come from various sources:

- Burns
- Infection
- Inflammation
- Arthritis
- Joint or muscle problems
- Pressure from a tumour
- Blockage of the stomach or intestine
- Surgical intervention.

Pain follows a complex pathway from the source of damage via sensory neurones to the brain. Pain receptors in the sensory nerves serve as a warning system, and a response via the motor nerves attempts to move the limb away from the pain. This nerve highway is made up of special pain receptors, which serve as a common pathway for pain information entering the central nervous system (CNS). These messages are like runners in a relay race: the nerves hand over the messages to other nerve cells in the spinal cord until they reach the brain, where they are interpreted.

- **A-delta fibres** transmit the initial pain sensation. These myelinated nerves send fast immediate messages from the site of injury, producing a sharp or tingling pain, like the pain felt when you hit your 'funny bone' (this being the site of your ulnar nerve). This also allows for localisation of pain.

Following this injury a second sensation, which is more like an ache, follows. This sensation is produced by the C-fibres.

- **C fibres** are unmyelinated fibres that carry the messages at a much slower pace, therefore the sensation felt is of a different quality, more like an ache.

These two important relays in the nervous system play a vital role in the pain experience. When you hit your 'funny bone', for example, the messages leave your elbow and reach the first relay station (A-delta fibres) situated in the spinal cord; they then cross over the midline of the spine and move along another pain fibre (C fibre) up to the subconscious brain – also known as pain gates. The message is then passed to the conscious brain, which evaluates the warning and reacts immediately; in this example, you feel that you have hit your elbow and you rub it to ease the pain.

Responses to pain

The body responds to pain in many ways. Physiological responses include raised blood pressure, tachycardia, increased respiration, dilation of the pupils and sweating. Behavioural responses include focusing on the pain, reporting pain, cries and moans, increased muscle tension and facial expression.

As pain continues and time passes, the body adapts to the stressors on it. The patient will then not report pain unless questioned. The patient may become physically inactive, or become quiet and sleep. The patient is adapting to pain. In a patient who is acutely ill, this phase can give a false impression of the patient's condition. Untreated pain can lead to complications. There are many reasons why pain should be treated:

- **Pulmonary complications:** The patient needs to be able to cough in order to clear secretions and ensure good gaseous exchange. This can be difficult if the diaphragm is splinted due to poor position or abdominal surgery. The inability to breathe can lead to pneumonia and sepsis, increasing the risk of death.

- **Cardiovascular function:** Pain can lead to increased stress, causing an increase in heart rate and blood pressure.

- **Mental state:** Good pain relief will impact on the patient's psychological state. It is humanitarian to control pain.

Treatments and interventions

Barriers to managing pain

Recent studies (Tycross, 2000; Lellan, 2004) show that often the hospital management of pain is still inadequate. Patients of all ages still experience pain during hospital admission, despite the wide range of analgesic drugs and techniques available. Various explanations for this have been proposed:

- **Lack of knowledge or interest in pain control:** This may be due to a lack of understanding of the nature of pain, lack of knowledge of analgesics, or lack of skill on the part of the prescriber to prescribe adequate or appropriate medication.

- **Failure to assess pain:** Earlier in the chapter the importance of pain assessment was discussed along with the need to assess effectiveness of the analgesia given. It is important that the nurse assesses the pain of all patients, even those who are quiet and mobile, as these may be the patients in greatest need of pain relief.

- **Failure to communicate:** It is important for patients to feel that they can communicate their need for analgesia to the nurse providing their care. When patients see that the nurse is busy, they are often reluctant to tell them of their pain, fearing that their need for analgesia will increase the nurse's workload. Patients should be able to feel that they can request analgesia at any time.

- **Fear of addiction and drug side-effects:** The fear of addiction often leads the medical and nursing profession to prescribe lower than optimal doses. It also leads to patients refusing medication, fearing that they may become 'addicted'. Communication with patients and clear explanations of how the drugs work can help to relieve anxieties in this area.

It is important to choose the correct route of administration. This will depend on the needs of the individual patient. The most suitable route for most patients is the oral route, but when swallowing is compromised, careful consideration should be given to an alternative route. The rectal route may be suitable, but this requires sensitive explanation and patient consent. Many medications come in liquid or soluble form and could therefore be administered via a nasogastric tube or jejunostomy tube, should one be in place; however, the nurse will need to consult local policy on the administration of medicine via these routes. *Table 8.2* shows some common routes of administration for various analgesic drugs.

Table 8.2: Common routes of administration for analgesic drugs

Route	Drug
Per rectum (PR)	Paracetamol – mild analgesic
	Diclofenac – NSAID (reduces inflammation)
Oral	Paracetamol
	Diclofenac
	Aspirin
	Codeine
	Dihydrocodeine
	Tramadol
	Morphine
Intramuscular (IM)	Morphine
	Tramadol
	Pethidine
Subcutaneous (SC)	Morphine
	Diamorphine
Transdermal	Fentanyl patch
Inhaled	Entonox
Epidural	Bupivacaine (local anaesthetic)
	Fentanyl (opiate)
Intravenous (IV)	Patient-controlled analgesia (PCA)
	Morphine
	Tramadol

Pain relief

Analgesic ladder

The analgesic ladder shown in *Figure 8.2* includes just a few of the common analgesics available. The British National Formulary (BNF) (Joint Formulary Committee, 2005) contains a larger range of analgesic drugs, allowing prescribers to select a drug according to the needs of the patient, taking into consideration any contraindications to their use in particular situations.

The choice of analgesic should be tailored to the individual patient, taking into consideration the following factors:

- **Patient preference:** Any known allergies or patient choice

- **Site and nature of the pain**

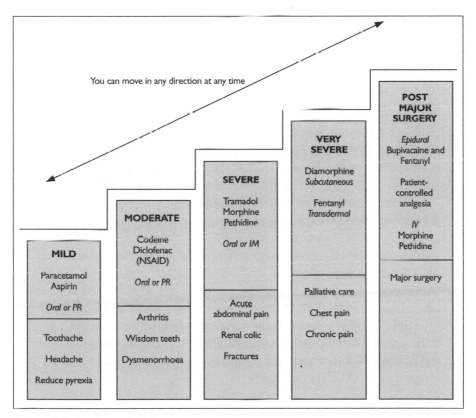

Figure 8.2: Analgesic ladder

- **Potential side-effects:** Many patients are reluctant to take analgesics because of the risk of constipation; if this is likely to be a problem, consider giving a laxative. Anti-emetics should also be considered if opiates are being administered.

- **Patient consent:** The patient's consent should be obtained before administering any analgesia, but particularly when an invasive procedure is involved, such as insertion of an epidural for postoperative pain management or labour, or a suppository via the rectal route.

The analgesic ladder works as a two-way process: as the pain increases, the patient climbs the ladder in terms of the analgesia required, and as the pain subsides, the patient comes down the ladder. An example would be the pain management of a patient who has had major abdominal surgery and leaves theatre with an epidural infusion running. This patient will start at the very top of the ladder, coming down as the pain subsides, adding in simple analgesia to maximise the analgesic effect. Remember that the patient would miss out the steps with the opiates if an opiate was already in the epidural bag, as additional systemic opiates could cause sedation and respiratory depression.

Routes of administration

- **Transdermal** patches may be appropriate for patients with long-term pain problems requiring strong analgesia. The patches are changed every 72 hours, and are convenient to use outside hospital as the patient does not have to worry about where he/she will be when it is time to take the medication. While this may not be the most common route for primary analgesia in the acutely ill adult, it may still be used in patients who are admitted wearing these patches for long-term problems.

- **Intramuscular** injections are another useful route of analgesic administration for acutely ill patients in hospital; however, the patient's skin condition and how long these methods can be sustained need to be taken into consideration. One drawback with controlled drugs given by injection, or by any route, is the need for two registered practitioners to be present at the time of administration; this can sometimes delay the administration of analgesia, causing the patient to be in pain for a longer period (Middleton, 2004).

Following surgical procedures, epidural analgesia or intravenous patient-controlled analgesia is widely used.

- **Epidural analgesia** is a method of blocking nerve roots lying within the epidural space. A fine plastic tube is inserted into the epidural space by an anaesthetist. A mixture of local anaesthetic (bupivacaine) and strong opiate (fentanyl) is given to provide optimum analgesia. With this route of analgesia, there is a need for close nursing observations and formal written guidelines for safe monitoring agreed by the hospital trust (Pain Society, 2002). Registered nurses who care for patients receiving epidural analgesia usually have to undergo a formal study day and an assessment of competency post-registration to enable them to carry out this extended role (Cox, 2001). Specialist nurses trained in pain management within the hospital environment form part of the acute pain service, which assesses the effectiveness of epidural analgesia in every patient receiving this form of analgesia, maintaining standards of care and offering support to ward staff (Mackrodt, 2001). The same support is offered to patients using patient-controlled analgesia (intravenous morphine).

- **Patient-controlled analgesia (PCA)** is a technique that allows the patient to self-administer prescribed amounts of morphine intravenously via a device attached to his/her arm. The patient uses a button to administer the doses (usually 1mg) around a lockout time (usually 5 minutes). Again, close nursing observations and guidelines are required, to enable monitoring of the effectiveness of the analgesia and the occurrence of side-effects, such as nausea, vomiting, hallucinations and pruritus.

- **Inhaled** entonox (50% nitrous oxide and 50% oxygen) is a well-established analgesic gas, commonly used during labour and by the ambulance service. It is self-administered and allows the patient to control when the pain relief takes place. Entonox can also be used in clinical practice for procedural pain, such as dressing changes, drain removal or physiotherapy, but the list is endless. It takes effect in approximately 20 seconds and the effect wears off very quickly. There are few side-effects and it is quick and simple to use.

Pain management services

In order for pain management to be effective, it is recommended that education and training in this vast specialty needs to take place (Pain Society, 2002). Specialist nurses in pain management help to support the nursing staff and offer advice on best practice. Pain is a unique phenomenon that is both physically and psychologically limiting for its duration (International Association of Pain, 1986; Carr, 1990; Melzack and Wall, 1991). The severity of the pain is also unique to each patient, and the coping strategies used are individual and tailored to the needs of the patient. The aim of reducing pain is the development of a carefully planned strategy, which can involve the pain team, the patient and the multidisciplinary team. The roles of both the acute pain team and the chronic pain team are still developing, with standards for best practice under continuous review. For the patient who is acutely ill, it is important to consider any chronic pain and continue to treat this, as well as any acute pain brought on by the patient's current condition.

Key learning points for *Chapter 8*

- Pain is what the patient says it is, and the patient should always be believed – believing the patient is the first step towards controlling the pain.
- Good patient history and pain assessment will provide a baseline for treatment and for assessing improvement.
- Regular basic observations and pain scoring will provide a continuous measure of the effectiveness of analgesia.
- Regular analgesia is more effective at controlling pain in the initial stages.
- Use the analgesic ladder as a guide to increasing analgesia when pain is severe and decreasing analgesia as pain improves.
- Treat the patient, not just the symptom.
- Pain control should be individual and tailored to the particular patient's needs.
- Providing good explanations of how the drugs work, and the alternatives if treatment is not sufficient, can help to relieve any anxieties that patients may have.
- Ensure regular administration of analgesia.
- Monitor patients for the side-effects of analgesia, and treat them as they occur:
  - If a patient feels sick – treat with an anti-emetic
  - If a patient feels that he/she is becoming constipated – consider a laxative.
- Consider the addition of non-pharmacological approaches to pain relief:
  - Transcutaneous electrical nerve stimulation (TENS)
  - Acupuncture
  - Relaxation.

Revision questions – pain management

1. What is pain?
2. Why is pain assessment so important?
3. Name four factors that need to be take into consideration when choosing a pain assessment tool for the acutely ill adult
4. How many different routes are there for administering morphine to an acutely ill adult?

Answers on page 202

References

Carr ECJ (1990) Postoperative pain: patients' experiences. *Journal of Advanced Nursing* **15**(1): 89–100

Carr ECJ, Thomas VJ (1997) Anticipating and experiencing postoperative pain: the patient's perspective. *Journal of Clinical Nursing* **16**(3): 191–201

Cox F (2001) Clinical care for patients with epidural infusions. *Professional Nurse* **16**(10): 1429–1432

Hunter D (1993) Acute pain. In: Carroll D, Bowsher D (1993) *Pain Management and Nursing Care*. Butterworth-Heinemann, Oxford

International Association of Pain (1986) Classification of chronic pain, description of chronic pain syndromes and definition of pain terms. *Pain* (Suppl 3)

Joint Formulary Committee (2004) *British National Formulary No. 50, September 2006*. British Medical Association and Royal Pharmaceutical Society of Great Britain, London

Lellan KM (2004) Postoperative pain: strategy for improving patient experiences. *Journal of Advanced Nursing* **46**(2): 179–185

Mackrodt K (2001) The role of the acute pain service. *British Journal of Perioperative Nursing* **11**(11): 492–497

Manias EM, Botti M, Bucknall T (2002) Observations of pain assessment and management – the complexities. *Journal of Clinical Practice* **11**(6): 724–733

Melzack RM, Wall P (1991) *The Challenge of Pain.* Penguin Books, London

Middleton C (2004) Barriers to the provision of effective pain management. *Nursing Times* **100**(3): 42–45

Pain Society (2002) *Recommendations for Nursing Practice in Pain Management.* Pain Society, London

Tycross A (2000) Educating nurses about pain management: the way forward. *Journal of Clinical Nursing* **11**(6): 705–714

CHAPTER 9

Transfer of the acutely ill adult

C Barclay

There are several reasons why an acutely ill patient in the ward environment may need to be transferred from one hospital to another (interhospital) or from one area to another within the same hospital (intrahospital):

- To facilitate diagnostic investigation that may determine a patient's management plan, eg. computed tomography (CT) scan or endoscopy
- To provide a higher level of care, eg. level 1, 2 or 3 (Department of Health, 2000)
- To undertake a surgical intervention
- To provide specialist services.

> **Additional learning point**
> Although the rationale for transfer may differ between patients, the overall aim should to be to minimise, where possible, the morbidity or mortality associated with transfer, thereby ensuring the best outcome for the patient.

The transfer of patients presents a challenging clinical scenario for the ward nurse, and the successful outcome of transfer relies on sound clinical judgment supported by a sensible management approach and appropriate delegation. The ward nurse needs to assess the clinical needs of the patient for transfer and consider which staff are appropriate to accompany the patient, taking into account the care requirements of the remaining patients on the ward.

Safe and effective transfer requires preparation of the patient, equipment and transfer personnel and, where clinically possible, resuscitation and stabilisation of the patient to ensure that the patient's physiological condition is not further compromised by the transfer process.

A variety of systematic approaches can be employed to ensure adequate preparation. One commonly used approach is the ACCEPT (**A**ssessment, **C**ontrol, **C**ommunication, **E**valuation, **P**reparation, **P**ackaging, **T**ransportation) methodology included in the Safe Transfer and Retrieval of Patients (StaR) manual developed by the Advanced Life Support Group (ALSG, 2002). Although normally applied to the inter/intrahospital transportation of intensive care patients, this type of systematic approach may be applied to any patient transfer to ensure appropriate preparation and consideration of all possible eventualities.

First phase – assessment and control

In the assessment phase it is essential that the patient's clinical condition is evaluated and the capabilities of the staff accompanying the patient are assessed. Within the ward environment, staffing issues may initially result in junior or untrained staff accompanying the patient. However, if the clinical skills of staff do not match the potential demands of the patient's current physiological condition, then patient and staff are potentially at risk; this may result in unnecessary critical incidents and further deterioration in the patient's condition.

Sometimes the urgency surrounding the transfer process is deemed the major priority, especially if the purpose of transfer is to facilitate diagnostic investigation that will determine subsequent treatment planning. However, if a patient's physiological condition deteriorates as a result of the transfer process, or results in cardiopulmonary arrest, then the investigation results are irrelevant. Definitive diagnosis on postmortem is of little use. It is imperative that the ward nurse, who is responsible for the patient's safety, takes an active part in the decision-making process. If necessary, any concerns should be discussed with the patient's senior clinicians and additional resuscitation measures instigated before transfer, even if this means delaying the investigation. At this point, consideration should be given to whether the patient and nurse should be accompanied by a member of the medical team.

If a patient is to be transferred to critical care for level 2 or 3 care, then a request for an anaesthetist or outreach nurse to accompany the patient, if there is concern about the patient's condition, is not unreasonable.

Additional learning point

It is important to remember that once a patient and nurse have left the confines of the ward environment, they have limited access to support services and need to be relatively self-sufficient. If their ability to do this is in doubt, the need for transfer should be reconsidered.

Key points to consider when asked to transfer a patient are:

- Is the patient's condition stable enough for transfer?
- Have you confirmed the clinical skills of the accompanying personnel?
- Do you need a medical member to accompany the patient on transfer?

Second phase – communication

Transferring a patient from one clinical area to another requires the involvement and coordination of several personnel. Good communication is the key to ensuring that these individuals work together as a cohesive team. Poor communication is often cited as one of the major causes of untoward incidents (Beckmann *et al*, 2004). To ensure that the receiving area is adequately prepared for the patient's arrival, the ward nurse must make sure that all information is communicated clearly, precisely and unambiguously. Communication begins in the assessment stage between all those involved in direct patient care.

- If the patient is to be transferred for investigation, eg. CT scan, communication is required between the scan personnel and the transfer nurse to prevent any delays once the patient has arrived in the radiology department, and to ensure that all the equipment required will be available.

- If the patient is to be transferred to a higher level of care, communication between the transfer nurse and intensive care staff is required to ensure bed availability and optimum timing of transfer, and to notify the receiving personnel of the patient's clinical condition and requirements to enable adequate preparation for the patient.

- If the patient is being transferred out of hospital, early communication between the transfer nurse and the ambulance team is necessary, specifying an appropriate time and the proposed location, outlining the patient's requirements during transfer, including equipment, eg. defibrillation, oxygen and suction.

Portering staff are a key consideration during all of these scenarios, and the level of communication with this important team should be given equal precedence to that of other disciplines. They will need to know where you are going, how many porters you need, your oxygen requirements and the mode of transport, eg. bed or stretcher.

The level and focus of communication will vary, depending on the needs of the patient and the personnel with whom you are communicating. However, during the communication process it is imperative that receiving staff are aware of the patient's clinical requirements and are adequately prepared to deal with them.

Successful communication has occurred when all relevant personnel have identified and understood all the information necessary to effect a safe patient transfer. The STaR manual (ALSG, 2002) recommends that the focus of communication should consist of:

- Who you are
- What is needed (from the listener)
- What are the relevant patient details
- What the problem is
- What has been done to address the problem
- What has happened.

While patient safety is paramount during the transfer process, time should be taken to inform relevant family members of the patient's condition, what is being done and why, and the potential risks involved. The transfer of acutely ill patients is associated with a degree of morbidity and mortality; the risks involved must be clearly explained. This can be undertaken by any member of the team who is aware of all the information concerning the patient.

Key points for the ward nurse to consider:

- Have you informed the necessary area of your requirements?
- Do you have the correct equipment?

Third phase – evaluation

The potential benefits for a patient who requires transfer from a ward environment to a level 2 or 3 area for specialist supportive measures are obvious. Difficulty arises when a patient whose condition is already unstable is being transferred for an investigative procedure: in this situation, consideration must be given to whether this is in the patient's best interest.

Evaluation of any clinical situation is a dynamic process and staff involved in the transfer situation should consider three key questions:

1. Do the benefits of transfer outweigh the associated risks?

For example, will taking a breathless patient on 100% oxygen for CT scan, and asking him/her to lie down, potentially cause the patient further respiratory problems? If the answer is yes, this should prompt the question: is this transfer appropriate? If the response from senior clinicians is yes, then control of the patient's airway before transfer needs to be considered or request the presence of an anaesthetist may be required.

2. Can the potential dangers of patient transportation be minimised by engaging experienced personnel?

For example, what is likely to go wrong, and do the transferring personnel possess skills to manage this situation? If the answer is no, then more qualified personnel or additional personnel, eg. medical staff, may be required.

3. Can adequate monitoring be maintained throughout the transfer process?

For example, what equipment is needed, are the transferring personnel familiar with the use of the equipment, and do they have everything they need to be able to deal with a likely emergency?

It must be remembered that once a patient and nurse have left the ward environment, there will be limited support. If, during the evaluation phase, there is any doubt about the availability of support, reassessment of whether this transfer is still appropriate is required.

Fourth phase – preparation and packaging

Preparation falls into three categories:

- Patient preparation
- Equipment preparation
- Personnel preparation.

Patient preparation

The aim of patient preparation is to ensure that the patient is in the best possible condition to withstand transfer. Using a systematic ABCDE approach, the ward nurse should be able to assess the patient's physiological condition and minimise foreseeable risks.

Airway

The questions that need to be asked here are:

- Is the airway patent?
- Is the airway secure?
- Is there potentially an airway problem?

Any concerns about the airway must be addressed with appropriate personnel. If there is any doubt that the patient will be able to maintain a patent airway, or concern regarding a fluctuating conscious level affecting the airway, then an assessment by an anaesthetist must be undertaken as intubation may be required.

Breathing

Most patients transferred from the ward area are likely to be self-ventilating, unless they have been intubated during a cardiopulmonary arrest, or elective intubation has been undertaken by the anaesthetist before transfer to a higher level of care. Any spontaneously breathing patient will need to be sat upright, where possible, and a non-breathing mask utilised during the transfer process unless clinically contraindicated, eg. patients who are reliant on hypoxic drive. If the patient has a chest drain in place, this should be properly secured and, where possible, a Heimlich valve drainage bag system or Heimlich valve alone should be in place. Clamps must accompany the patient in case of disconnection, but the chest drain should never be clamped, unless in an emergency.

Circulation

Establishment of secure venous access is mandatory. It is preferable to have at least one wide-bore intravenous (IV) cannula on either side of the patient. Attached to one of these should be a giving set with an appropriate colloid. Any routine IV fluids or medication should be discontinued for the duration of the transfer journey to prevent accidental disconnection and reduce unnecessary equipment. If the patient is on any medication that cannot be discontinued, the nurse must ensure that an appropriate amount of the relevant drug is available for the transfer process. This should be drawn up before the patient and nurse leave the ward.

Disability

If spinal immobilisation is required, this must be done with a hard cervical collar rather than saline bags. Staff skilled in moving these patients should also either accompany the patient or be available at the destination to enable transfer from bed to scanning machine or from bed to bed.

Exposure and environment

It is unlikely that patients will become hypothermic while being transferred intrahospital. However, consideration must be given to the fact that lifts and corridors within hospitals are cold environments; also, the dignity of the patient needs to be maintained at all times. If the patient is undergoing an ambulance transfer, he/she must be adequately wrapped to reduce the risk of heat loss.

Equipment preparation

Any equipment that accompanies the patient during the transfer must be rationalised to prevent clutter and panic by the transfer personnel, and the transfer personnel must be able to use the equipment and be familiar with it.

One of the most important considerations during transfer is correct calculation of the oxygen supply. This is based on the likely transfer time and the oxygen concentration and necessary flow rate being delivered to the patient. Flow rates necessary to obtain various oxygen targets through a Hudson mask or a non-rebreathe mask are identified in *Table 9.1*.

Table 9.1: Oxygen flow rates and percentages

Oxygen needed (%)	24	28	35	40	60	100
Delivery rate (litres/min)	2	4	8	10	12	15

Once the flow rate and the estimated journey time are known, the number of cylinders required to ensure an adequate oxygen supply can be calculated. It is always advisable to double the oxygen supply in case of any delay or problem with oxygen delivery. Always check your cylinders are full.

Oxygen requirement =
2 x estimated journey time (minutes) x flow rate (litres/min)
at the given percentage of oxygen

For example, patient A is going to CT: the estimated journey time is an hour and the patient is on 10 litres of oxygen/min. Using the above formula, the oxygen requirement is therefore:

2 x 60 minutes x 10 litres/min = 1200 litres

So, a minimum of a size F (or equivalent small cylinder) cylinder will be needed for the transfer. Oxygen cylinder capacities are shown in *Table 9.2*.

Table 9.2: Oxygen cylinder capacities

Cylinder size	Capacity
D	340 litres
E	680 litres
F	1360 litres

Any unstable or acutely ill patient must be monitored during the transfer process. This must include ECG, oxygen saturations and either invasive or non-invasive monitoring of blood pressure; in the ward environment, blood pressure is likely to be monitored by non-invasive methods. In these circumstances, it is also essential to take with you a self-filling Ambu bag with reservoir and oxygen tubing, an arrest box and spare bag of colloid, and any necessary medications.

Personnel preparation

As stated previously, it is important that staff accompanying the patient are able to deal with any likely eventuality; therefore, if the patient is acutely unwell and unstable it may be prudent to have either medical or experienced nursing staff accompany the patient. They must be able to use the equipment that is available to them, and be able to instigate basic life support measures, should the need arise.

Packaging

When packaging the patient before transfer it is important that all lines and leads from monitors are adequately secured to prevent them falling out or being pulled out. Infusions and drains should be adequately secured to prevent disconnection and any equipment taken on the transfer should be appropriately placed on the bed or the stretcher – not on top of the patient. At this point it is worth remembering that any notes, X-rays and investigation request forms should accompany the patient.

Transportation

Most acutely ill patients within the ward environment who are being transferred for either investigation or a higher level of care are normally transferred on their own bed. Before leaving the ward, the nurse should ensure that:

- All necessary equipment is available
- Personnel are ready
- Oxygen cylinders are present
- Notes and X-rays are available
- A final re-evaluation of the patient's condition has been carried out.

Are you still happy to leave? If the answer is yes:

* Contact the receiving area to inform the staff that you are on your way.

It is also beneficial to have a member of staff go ahead of the transfer to locate lifts and evacuate members of the public to enable smooth transition.

Key learning points for *Chapter 9*

- Systematic preparation will optimise patient safety.

- Remember the ACCEPT acronym (Assessment, Control, Communication, Evaluation, Preparation and packaging, Transportation).

- Oxygen cylinders are available in different sizes; be sure you know the capacity of the cylinder you are taking.

- It is important to call ahead to your destination so that the receiving team is ready for your arrival.

- Have you considered the benefits of moving the patient against the possible risks of transfer? The benefits must be greater than the risks if the transfer is to be successful.

- If you are not confident that you can maintain patient safety, ask for more senior help.

- Remember that transfer is not complete until either you have returned to the ward environment following an investigative procedure, or you have safely handed over the patient to the receiving team. This involves an effective handover of the management of all clinical requirements, any events that occurred during transfer and present condition of the patient. Before the transfer can be considered complete, the relatives have to be informed of the patient's arrival back on the ward or on the receiving unit.

Revision question – patient transfer

Case scenario

A 56-year-old woman admitted with pancreatitis to your ward yesterday requires a CT scan to establish the cause of the disease process and assist with treatment planning. She weighs 75kg and her latest observations are:

- Heart rate 120 beats/min, irregular
- Blood pressure 89/40mmHg (normal systolic 120mmHg)
- Respiratory rate 32 breaths/min
- Temperature 38°C
- Urine output 20ml in last hour
- Oxygen saturation 92% on 40% oxygen

She has an intravenous infusion in situ running at 125ml/h, through which morphine patient-controlled analgesia is being delivered for pain relief. The porter has arrived to take the patient to CT. You are the nurse in charge of the ward:

1. What would you do?
2. What actions need to take place before this patient can be transferred?
3. Whom would you request to accompany this patient?
4. How would you evaluate whether the patient is fit for transfer?

Answers on page 203

References

Advanced Life Support Group (ALSG) (2002) *Safe Transfer and Retrieval: The Practical Approach*. BMJ Books, London

Beckmann U, Gillies DM, Berenholtz SM *et al* (2004) Incidents relating to the intra-hospital transfer of critically ill patients. An analysis of the reports submitted to the Australian Incident Monitoring Study in Intensive. *Intensive Care Medicine* **30**(8): 1579–1585

Department of Health (2000) *Comprehensive Critical Care: A review of adult critical care services* (2000) HMSO, London

Bibliography

British National Formulary No. 50 (September 2005) British Medical Association and Royal Pharmaceutical Society of Great Britain, London

Bennett P, Brown MJ (1993) *Clinical Pharmacology*. 9th edn. Churchill Livingstone, London

Kumar P, Clark M (Eds) (2005) *Clinical Medicine*. 6th edn. WB Saunders, Edinburgh

Hudak C, Gallo B, Goncemortin P (1998) *Critical Care Nursing: A holistic approach*. Raven, Philadelphia

Mosby's Medical, Nursing & Allied Health Dictionary (2002) 6th edn. Mosby, St Louis

Schell HM, Puntillo KA (2001) *Critical Care Nursing Secrets*. Hanley and Belfus, Philadelphia

Sheppard M, Wright M (Eds) (2000) *Principles and Practice of High Dependency Nursing*. 1st edn. Baillière Tindall, Edinburgh

Torrance C, Serginson E (1997) *Surgical Nursing*.12th edn. Baillière Tindall, London

Tortora G, Grabowski S (2003) *Principles of Anatomy and Physiology*. 10th edn. Wiley & Sons Inc., New York

Wilson K, Waugh A (2001) *Ross and Wilson Anatomy and Physiology in Health and Illness*. 9th edn. Churchill Livingstone

Appendixes

Appendix 1: Modified early warning scoring (MEWS) system flow pathway

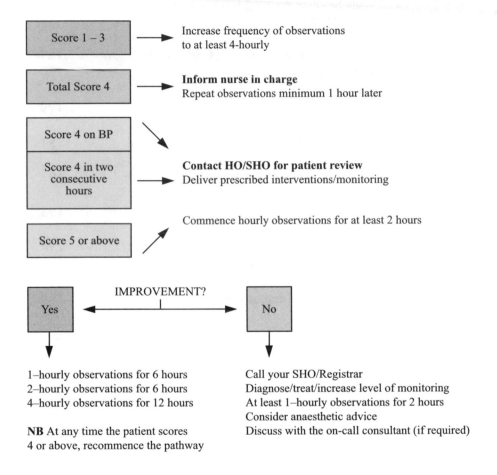

| Score 1 – 3 | → | Increase frequency of observations to at least 4-hourly |

| Total Score 4 | → | **Inform nurse in charge** Repeat observations minimum 1 hour later |

Score 4 on BP

Score 4 in two consecutive hours → **Contact HO/SHO for patient review** Deliver prescribed interventions/monitoring

Commence hourly observations for at least 2 hours

Score 5 or above

IMPROVEMENT?

Yes ← → No

1–hourly observations for 6 hours
2–hourly observations for 6 hours
4–hourly observations for 12 hours

NB At any time the patient scores
4 or above, recommence the pathway

Call your SHO/Registrar
Diagnose/treat/increase level of monitoring
At least 1–hourly observations for 2 hours
Consider anaesthetic advice
Discuss with the on-call consultant (if required)

Printed with permission of the UHL Critical Care outreach team

Appendix 2: Assessment of a patient for CPAP or high-flow oxygen therapy

(ABGs = arterial blood gases; BP = blood pressure; CVS = cardiovascular system)

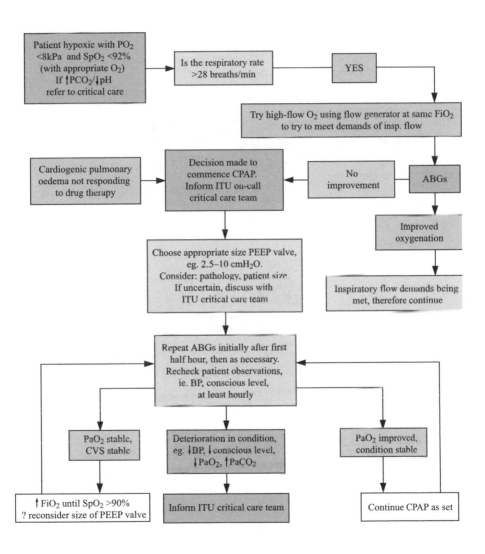

Patient hypoxic with PO_2 <8kPa and SpO_2 <92% (with appropriate O_2) If $\uparrow PCO_2/\downarrow pH$ refer to critical care

Is the respiratory rate >28 breaths/min

YES

Try high-flow O_2 using flow generator at same FiO_2 to try to meet demands of insp. flow

Cardiogenic pulmonary oedema not responding to drug therapy

Decision made to commence CPAP. Inform ITU on-call critical care team

No improvement

ABGs

Improved oxygenation

Choose appropriate size PEEP valve, eg. 2.5–10 cmH_2O. Consider: pathology, patient size If uncertain, discuss with ITU critical care team

Inspiratory flow demands being met, therefore continue

Repeat ABGs initially after first half hour, then as necessary. Recheck patient observations, ie. BP, conscious level, at least hourly

PaO_2 stable, CVS stable

Deterioration in condition, eg. $\downarrow$BP, $\downarrow$conscious level, $\downarrow PaO_2$, $\uparrow PaCO_2$

PaO_2 improved, condition stable

$\uparrow FiO_2$ until SpO_2 >90% ? reconsider size of PEEP valve

Inform ITU critical care team

Continue CPAP as set

Appendix 3: Weaning from CPAP

Weaning a patient from a continuous positive airways system (CPAP) system needs to be done slowly with close observation at each step, as shown below (PEEP = positive end-expiratory pressure).

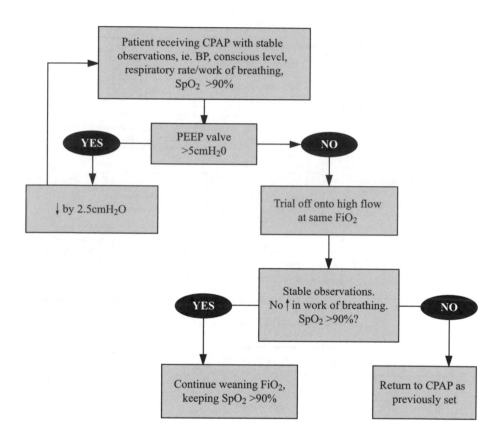

Appendix 4: Assessing postoperative respiratory failure

Does the patient have these RISK FACTORS?
Elderly or obese patient
Pre-existing cardiopulmonary disease, smoker
Major abdominal or thoracic surgery
Exercise limited to a flight of stairs or less

Does the patient exhibit these IMPORTANT SIGNS?
Respiratory rate (RR) >30 breaths/min
SpO$_2$ <90% on air   Drowsy/confused, pain
Temperature   Productive cough
Added sounds in chest or reduced air entry

The patient requires these BASELINE INVESTIGATIONS
Chest X-ray   12-lead ECG
Arterial blood gases   Sputum and blood culture
Full blood count   Urea and electrolytes

Your nursing care should include these GENERAL MEASURES
Sit patient up   Give OXYGEN   Physiotherapy
Pain control   Monitoring of RR and SpO$_2$
Reassurance   Tissues and sputum pot
CONSIDER THE CAUSE and be prepared

Splinted diaphragm (atelectasis, pain, distended abdomen)
Pulmonary oedema (left ventricular fibrillation, fluid overload, ARDS)
Nosocomial pneumonia

Hypoventilation (eg. opioid narcosis)
Pneumothorax
Exacerbation of lung disease
Pulmonary embolus (PE)
Compensation for metabolic acidosis

May benefit from use of **facial continuous positive airways pressure (CPAP)**
Diuretics only if evidence of pulmonary oedema
Antibiotics

Narcosis: Naloxone 0.1–0.8mg IV
Pneumothorax: Consider chest drain
Wheeze: Bronchodilators
Pulmonary embolus: Thrombolyse/Anticoagulant
Acidosis: Consider sepsis ?cause

Indications for admission to higher level of care
Increased level of observations and nursing input required.
Facial CPAP or ventilation

Printed with permission of the UHL Critical Care outreach team

Appendix 5: Does your patient have sepsis? Step-by-step

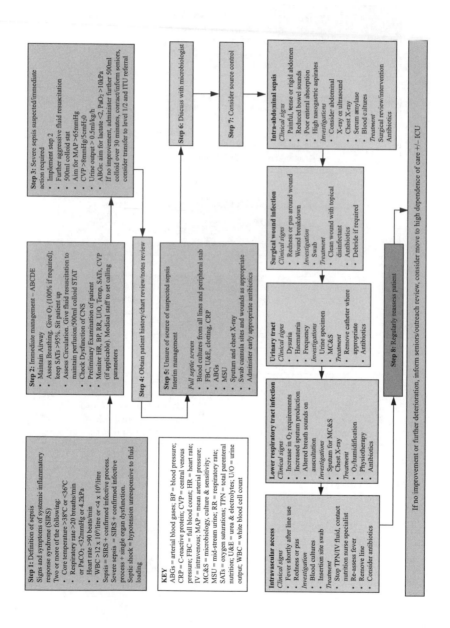

Printed with permission of the UHL Critical Care outreach team

Appendix 6: CPAP prescription and monitoring chart

Please affix patient label

WARD _____
Prescribed start date: _____
Diagnosis: _____
Prescribed _____

Critical care on-call team informed   YES [ ]   NO [ ]

	Pre-CPAP								
Time									
Prescribed PEEP									
Signature Dr									
FIO_2									
SaO_2									
Heart rate									
Blood pressure									
Respiratory rate									
Safety valve in situ									
Prescribed valve working									
H_2O heater temperature									
Facial pressure areas checked									
Signature									

Discontinued _____   Date/Time

Appendix 7: Summary of nursing care needs for patients receiving parenteral nutrition

	Rationale	Frequency	Action
Fluid balance chart	To monitor hydration	Constantly	Measure daily input/output. Observe for thirst, lethargy, low urine output, ankle oedema/ postural hypotension or breathlessness
Weight	To monitor hydration state	Twice weekly on Monday and Thursday	Weigh Monday and Thursday (in similar clothing, at same time of day, on same scales). Record weight
Blood glucose	To ensure that patient tolerates glucose load of feed	4-hourly for first 72 hours, then twice daily if STABLE	BM Stix 4-hourly for first 72 hours. If patient stable, reduce frequency. (Consider) sliding scale insulin if BM shows blood glucose >12mmol consistently
Temperature pulse and respiration	To detect signs of infection/line malposition (tachyarrhythmia may show line malposition)	4-hourly	Monitor 4-hourly while on parenteral nutrition
Line entry and dressing sites	To detect signs of localised infection (warmth, redness, tenderness, exudate and swelling)	Observe catheter entry/exit site daily	Observe site(s) daily for discharge by removing dressing and replacing with sterile dressing using an aseptic technique. Review as part of full clinical condition review

Appendix 8: Answers to revision questions

Chapter 1

1. *Priorities for assessing Mr Peters*

   A.   Is he maintaining his own airway?
   B.   Is he breathing? What is his respiratory rate? Is it shallow? What is his oxygen saturation? Is he receiving oxygen?
   C.   What is his blood pressure? Is it lower or higher than normal? What is his pulse? Is it regular? Is it fast or slow?

   Maintaining Mr Peter's safety is crucial – once you have done A, B and C, you can assess him further. You need to treat any adverse signs that you find, eg. low blood pressure, low oxygen saturation. Seek senior help if in doubt.

   You need to observe his wound and check his temperature; pain relief should be administered as prescribed.

   When you have carried out any treatments required, you need to reassess the patient to check for improvement or deterioration.

2. *Early warning scores*

a.	HR = 0	Urine = 0	
	RR = 1	Temp = 0	
	BP = 0	Neuro = 0	EWS = 1
b.	HR = 1	Urine = 1	
	RR = 2	Temp = 0	
	BP = 0	Neuro = 0	EWS = 4
c.	HR = 2	Urine = 1	
	RR = 2	Temp = 0	
	BP = 0	Neuro = 1	EWS = 6
d.	HR = 0	Urine = 2	
	RR = 1	Temp = 0	
	BP = 0	Neuro = 1	EWS = 4

Chapter 2

1. *Priorities for assessing Mr Smith*

   A. Is he maintaining his own airway?
   B. Is he breathing? What is his respiratory rate? Is it shallow? What is his oxygen saturation? Is he receiving any oxygen?
   C. What is his blood pressure? Is it lower or higher than normal? What is his pulse? Is it regular? Is it fast or slow?

   Maintaining Mr Smith's safety is crucial – once you have done A, B and C, you can assess him further. You need to treat any adverse signs you find, eg. low blood pressure, low oxygen saturation. Seek senior help if in doubt.

   You need to observe his wound and check his temperature; pain relief should be administered as prescribed.

   When you have carried out any treatments required, you need to reassess him to check for improvement or deterioration.

   Maintain good hydration to ensure that Mr Smith's secretions remain loose and it is easy for him to expectorate. Encourage deep breathing, and ask the physiotherapist to see him.

   It may be necessary to check arterial blood gases to ensure that Mr Smith is not retaining carbon dioxide and his oxygenation is greater than 8kPa. If not, he will require supplementary humidified oxygen.

   Blood pressure, heart rate and respiratory rate need to be monitored on an ongoing basis.

2. You should consider the possibility that Mrs Jones has sepsis, and take steps to identify the source. The wound would be the most obvious source, but other possible sites of infection should be excluded. A step-by-step guide to assessing your patient for sepsis is shown in *Appendix 5*.

Chapter 3

1. ***Figure 3.13*** = ventricular fibrillation
   Call cardiac arrest and start resuscitation; early defibrillation is needed.

   Figure 3.14 = sinus rhythm
   Check your patient: if he/she is alert with a good blood pressure, no action related to cardiac rhythm is needed.

   Figure 3.15 = first-degree heart block
   Check your patient: this rhythm is generally a stable rhythm and no action is needed.

2. ***Which nerve supplies the sino-atrial node in the heart?***
   The vagus nerve.

3. ***Why are patients with atrial fibrillation given anticoagulation?***
   Because they have an increased risk of thrombus formation.

4. ***Where is the external pacemaker kept in your hospital?***
   Check your own hospital for this.

Chapter 4

1. ***What is the maximum score that can be achieved using the Glasgow Coma Scale?***
   15

2. ***What is the priority in an unconscious patient?***
   Maintaining an adequate airway.

3. ***Name the three meninges of the brain.***
   Pia mater, dura mater and arachnoid mater.

4. ***What is the most common antibiotic regimen used to treat bacterial meningitis?***
   Ceftriaxone 4g stat dose and then once daily ceftriaxone 2g.
   Benzylpenicillin 1.2g can be given if no other antibiotics are available.

Chapter 5

1. **What nursing interventions will you carry out?**
   - Check the volume of urine in the catheter and then empty the catheter; divide the volume (135ml) by the number of hours since midnight. This is likely to be <0.5ml/kg per hour.
   - Put Mr Jones back onto a fluid balance chart.
   - Omit lisinopril – inform medical staff.

2. **When will you next complete a set of observations?**
   Check observations now and in one hour's time.

3. **What are your initial concerns?**
   Establish Mr Jones' fluid balance status.

4. **What other information will you want to collect?**
   - You could check a urinalysis for specific gravity to see whether Mr Jones' urine is concentrated.
   - You could check his blood results to see if the urea level is elevated.
   - You should be concerned that his possible hypovolaemia is causing pre-renal failure.

Chapter 6

1. **Why do patients with abdominal pain have an increased risk of developing respiratory failure?**
   Patients with abdominal pain develop splinting of the diaphragm, and so do not expand their lung bases, resulting in atelectasis of the lower lobes.

2. **What is the pH in the stomach?**
   Between pH 3 and 4 (Metheny *et al*, 1994).

3. **Give the three main causes of pancreatitis.**
   Alcohol abuse, gallstones and viral infections.

4. **Give two ways of measuring abdominal distension.**
   Bladder pressure and girth measurements.

Metheney NA *et al* (1994) pH testing of feeding tube aspirates to determine placement. *Nutrition in Clinical Practice* **9**: 185–190

Chapter 7

1. ***Why is nutrition important?***
   Undernourished patients show physiological dysfunction that results in muscular weakness, impaired immunity and reduced wound healing. Specifically, nutritional support aims to reduce infection, wound breakdown, fatigue and neurological, psychological, cardiac, respiratory, gastrointestinal, endocrine and functional impairment.

   Prospective randomised controlled trials of nutritional support improved outcome in general (eg. management of undernutrition-related complications associated with longer hospital stay, re-admission, morbidity and mortality) and in disease-specific patient groups.

   Mortality is directly related to the degree of malnutrition experienced. Undernourished patients require more intensive nursing than normally nourished patients with similar underlying clinical problems, have a longer hospital stay with more complications, a higher re-admission rate, and higher morbidity and mortality, especially from sepsis.

2. ***When should the acutely ill patient be fed?***
   Early postoperative enteral feeding is a valid alternative to parenteral feeding in patients undergoing major surgery. Immediate postoperative enteral feeding in patients undergoing intestinal resection is safe (Bengmark *et al*, 2001), prevents an increase in gut mucosal permeability and produces a positive nitrogen balance. Feeding within 6 hours of insult can improve the hormonal response to stress, improve wound healing and decrease the incidence of bowel obstruction and septic complications.

Bengmark S, Andersson R, Mangiante G (2001) Uninterrupted perioperative enteral nutrition. *Clinical Nutrition* **20**(1): 11–19

3. ***Why is it important to ascertain the position of a nasogastric tube before use, and how can the position of the tube be determined accurately?***
   Perforation, intracranial penetration, tracheobronchial intubation (risk 0.9–2.4%), tracheopleural intubation through intact artificial airways, pneumothorax and failure to advance due to coiling of the tube in the mouth, either in front of the teeth or under the tongue, have been reported in association with nasogastric tube insertion. There

may be serious adverse consequences of feeding through a tube that is malpositioned. A malpositioned tube most commonly enters the trachea, bronchus or lung (usually right lung). Feeding through a tube into the lung may result in aspiration pneumonia and/or death.

Once the nasogastric tube has advanced to the required length, its position should be checked by aspirating gastric residual and testing its pH with indicator paper. If the pH is <5.5 (National Patient Safety Agency [NPSA], 2005), it is safe to administer feed, fluid or medication via the tube.

Nasogastric tube position should be checked before starting feed, before re-commencing use of the tube after a rest period or bag change, and if there is any possibility of tube dislodgement.

In patients for whom an aspirate is unobtainable, or who have an aspirate with pH >5.5, a chest X-ray may be necessary to confirm the correct positioning of a nasogastric tube. The X-ray is only conclusive at the time it is taken, as the tube may move with vomiting, retching, coughing, pulling or patient movement.

National Patient Safety Agency (NPSA) (2005) How to confirm the correct position of nasogastric feeding tubes in infants, children and adults. Available at: http://www.npsa.nhs.uk/site/media/documents/857_Insert-finalWeb.pdf (last accessed 17.01.06)

4. *Is auscultation an effective method of checking nasogastric tube position?*
No. It is unsafe because of the risk of hearing transmitted bowel sounds, and it may only be 60% reliable.

5. *What is the indication for PEG placement?*
The acutely ill patient with a functional gastrointestinal tract who is likely to require long-term nutritional support (>6 weeks).

6. *What complications may arise from PEG placement and feed administration?*
Aspiration pneumonia, subcutaneous abscess, gastric or bowel perforation, gastric haemorrhage, gastro-colic fistula, wound dehiscence, tube blockage/malfunction, tube dislodgement, peristomal infection (approx 6%), cellulitis and peritonitis (approx 1%).

7. *What are the indications for parenteral nutrition?*
Patients with acute or chronic intestinal failure due to reduced intestinal absorption require macronutrient and/or water and electrolyte

supplements to maintain health and/or growth (Nightingale, 2001).
If the amount of enteral nutrition absorbed is insufficient to meet the
patient's requirements or the administration of enteral nutrition is
contraindicated by the patient's condition, parenteral nutrition is the
route of choice for nutritional support.

Nightingale JMD (2001) Definition and classification of intestinal failure.
In: Nightingale JMD (Ed) *Intestinal Failure*. Greenwich Medical
Media, London

8. *What are the complications of parenteral nutrition line insertion
   and feed administration?*
   The most common complication is pneumothorax. Other insertion-
   related complications include line malposition, venous or arterial
   puncture with consequent extravasation and haematoma, and damage
   to nerves or the thoracic ducts. Once in situ, the most common
   complication is catheter-related sepsis. Catheter occlusion or
   dislodgement, hyperglycaemia, rebound hypoglycaemia, deficiencies of
   potassium, sodium, phosphate, zinc, magnesium, trace elements, folate,
   essential fatty acids and vitamins and hepatic disturbances, including
   elevated liver enzymes, fatty infiltration, jaundice and intrahepatic
   cholestasis, may also occur.

9. *What are the risk factors for parenteral nutrition line-related sepsis?*
   * The use of multi-lumen lines as opposed to dedicated single-
     lumen lines
   * The material from which the line is constructed.
   * Increased number of connections between the parenteral nutrition
     administration set and the patient's central venous access device
   * Increased number of manipulations of the line
   * Subcutaneous tunnelling of the line at insertion may prolong
     catheter life but have equivocal benefit in the management of
     catheter-related sepsis.
   * The skill, training and experience of the person manipulating
     the line.
   * For management of suspected line infection (see *Table 7.2*).

10. *What monitoring is required for patients receiving parenteral
    nutrition?*
    On an ongoing basis, the team caring for the patient receiving
    parenteral nutrition need to ensure that it is an appropriate treatment.
    To assess suitability, one needs to ascertain whether the patient's

gastrointestinal tract is functional, the patient's current nutritional status, the patient's current clinical condition, and whether the patient's nutritional status is likely to be affected by any (proposed) treatment, investigation or ongoing sepsis.

Regular blood tests are required for patients being considered for parenteral nutrition, and as ongoing assessment while they are receiving it. *Table 7.1* lists the tests recommended for patients before they receive parenteral nutrition and during the time they are receiving it.

Specific nursing care needs of patients receiving parenteral nutrition are summarised in *Appendix 7*.

Chapter 8

1. *What is pain?*
   Pain is complex and unique to each individual patient. It is an emotion that causes unpleasant stress on the body; it should therefore be treated, however small.

2. *Why is pain assessment so important?*
   Pain assessment, using a pain assessment tool, is important because it is the initial step towards pain control: it identifies the location of the pain, how long it has been there, and what type of pain the patient is experiencing. [Q reworded so that it answers the question - ?OK]

3. *Name four factors that need to be taken into consideration when choosing a pain assessment tool for the acutely ill adult.*
   Simple and easy to understand, appropriate to the patient group, reliable and valid.

4. *How many different routes are there for administering morphine to an acutely ill adult?*
   Four: oral, intramuscular, subcutaneous and intravenous (via bolus or PCA machine) routes.

Chapter 9

1. *What would you do?*
    Contact medical staff and explain your concerns about the patient's cardiovascular and respiratory status, ie. low blood pressure, low urine output and tachycardia, increased respiratory rate and suitability for transfer.

2. *What actions need to take place before this patient can be transferred?*
    Medical assessment and fluid resuscitation.

3. *Whom would you request to accompany this patient?*
    Medical and nursing staff.

4. *How would you evaluate whether the patient is fit for transfer?*
    Reassess the effectiveness of medical interventions on the patient's condition, ie. are blood pressure, urine output and heart rate improving?

Index